PRAISE F
MORE THAN A MOM

"*More Than a Mom* epitomizes everything I love about Kari Kampakis and the way she uses her voice to speak wisdom and truth that goes straight to your heart. As moms it can be so easy to lose ourselves in the daily grind, and Kari's words are so encouraging. This book is a must-read for everyone who's doing their best to raise strong, Godly kids in a world that is constantly trying to beat you down. Kari is refreshing, honest, and real. Every page of this book is like hearing from a dear friend who is assuring you it's all going to be okay, and you are up for the challenges that come with motherhood."

MELANIE SHANKLE, *NEW YORK TIMES*
BESTSELLING AUTHOR AND SPEAKER

"Kari Kampakis has done it again with *More Than a Mom*. With compassion, honesty, and vulnerability, Kari encourages moms to take a holistic look at their own wellness in all the ways that matter most. This book is beautifully researched and written—with relatable stories from Kari's life as well as from other moms—and I walked away from it feeling inspired, understood, and comforted. What a timely reminder that we will ultimately best care for our families when we prioritize caring for ourselves. Reading *More Than a Mom* feels like spending time with a trusted friend, and I have no doubt that moms of all ages and stages will be uplifted by Kari's words."

SOPHIE HUDSON, BESTSELLING AUTHOR AND
CO-HOST OF *THE BIG BOO CAST*

"In marathon running and training, 'hitting the wall' is when your muscles and strength give out despite your will. I had long associated this term with sports—until I hit the wall as a mom. Despite my will, I could no longer keep an intense pace, and denying myself the dignity of self-care and proper rest landed me in the hospital, and it took a surgery to find rest for my soul. That health scare seven years ago shook my world in the best way as it highlighted how my well-being directly correlates to how well I can serve my family. In *More Than a Mom*, Kari offers wisdom and encouragement to help us avoid hitting that same wall. She fuels us with reminders that we are children of God, He cares for us, and He desires that we care for ourselves so that we can care for the children and the precious family He has entrusted to us. Don't hit the wall like I did. Instead, read this book."

ELISABETH HASSELBECK, *NEW YORK TIMES* BESTSELLING AUTHOR, DAYTIME EMMY AWARD WINNER, AND AUTHOR OF THE CHILDREN'S BOOK *FLASHLIGHT NIGHT: AN ADVENTURE IN TRUSTING GOD*

"For the first ten years of motherhood, I ran myself ragged. I never got enough sleep, and I was constantly exhausted, stressed, and running on fumes. Only when I hit rock bottom and crashed did I finally realize that not prioritizing my health and well-being hurt everyone. In *More Than a Mom*, Kari Kampakis inspires moms with practical ways to start making their emotional, physical, and spiritual health a priority. Every mom can benefit from reading this book and taking it to heart! I only wish I had it around eighteen years ago when I first became a mom!"

CRYSTAL PAINE, *NEW YORK TIMES* BESTSELLING AUTHOR, BLOGGER, PODCASTER, AND BIOLOGICAL/FOSTER/ADOPTIVE MOM OF SIX

"Kari's writing never fails to feel like a handwritten note from a close friend, which makes her latest book especially wonderful. Kari identifies the often unacknowledged or overlooked needs we have as moms, affirms the significance of us tending to our own souls as we tend to the precious souls God has entrusted to us, and shows us how to model healthy and biblical self-care to our kids. Much needed renewal awaits you in these pages!"

JEANNIE CUNNION, BESTSELLING AUTHOR OF
DON'T MISS OUT AND *MOM SET FREE*

"I have long admired Kari and her passion for helping moms be the best version of themselves they can be. In *More Than a Mom*, Kari shares the lessons she's learned through her journey in motherhood and reminds us that we all struggle. This book will keep you inspired to take care of your own soul first, in order to empower your kids. Because at the end of the day, we are all more than a mom."

MICHELE BORBA, ED.D, AUTHOR OF *THRIVERS: THE SURPRISING REASONS WHY SOME KIDS STRUGGLE AND OTHERS SHINE*

"Both mothers and grandmothers will be inspired by this gracious wisdom. In an age of social media that leaves us constantly questioning our mothering skills and feeling inadequate, it's a refreshing reminder of what it means to be human as we raise and shape the next generation. *More Than a Mom* is brilliantly written, and an essential read to overcome a culture of parent-shaming and self-doubt. This book is a true gift for all moms."

SUE SCHEFF, AUTHOR OF *SHAME NATION: THE GLOBAL EPIDEMIC OF ONLINE HATE*

"Kari's authentic voice and practical approach have been helping moms parent better for years. Now, in *More Than a Mom*, Kari helps us give our kids one of the things they need the very most: a healthy mom! With vulnerability, compassion, and hard-earned wisdom, Kari has created a guidebook that can benefit every mom."

MONICA SWANSON, AUTHOR OF *BOY MOM* AND HOST OF *THE BOY MOM PODCAST*

MORE THAN A MOM

MORE THAN
A MOM

How Prioritizing Your Wellness Helps
You (and Your Family) Thrive

KARI KAMPAKIS

W PUBLISHING GROUP

AN IMPRINT OF THOMAS NELSON

To my sisters in motherhood. I pray this book encourages you and reminds you that you are loved, needed, and worthy of care and attention.

CONTENTS

CONTENTS

INTRODUCTION

Don't confuse invisibility with insignificance.

CHRISTINE CAINE[1]

The day I became a mom was the best day of my life. I had no idea what a game-changer meeting my baby would be.

I was physically exhausted from labor, yet mentally elated. Who knew that my heart could swell with such unconditional, unreciprocated, one-way love? I knew that my daughter would never love me the way I loved her, yet that was the beauty of our situation. After a lifetime of selfishness, I was ready to be the Giver. And I was determined to do it well.

Then and there, my life split into two: *Before* and *After*. If ever I had questioned my existence, or wondered what good I added to this world, I finally had an answer. God had chosen me to raise this remarkable child, and she inspired in me a sense of purpose unlike anything I had known before.

In many ways, motherhood was a dream, even with the sleep deprivation and worry. I saw the world through new eyes, the eyes of a protective mom. I marveled over the love for my child that felt simultaneously tender and fierce.

Days turned into weeks, weeks turned into years, and years turned into seasons as my baby grew up and welcomed three siblings. Each new child evoked a new rush of elation and extra determination to do motherhood well.

I can't pinpoint when motherhood started to feel hard because every stage has brought trials and challenges. What I can say now, twenty years into this journey, is that it has surpassed my greatest expectations—and dashed some expectations too.

Motherhood has brought countless moments of joy, laughter, transformation, meaning, gratitude, and euphoria. It has convinced me that there is, indeed, a heaven and a God who created us and loves us all. But on the hard days, there are struggles behind the scenes, struggles that we talk about only with our closest friends because we need someone who understands.

I'm talking about those moments when we feel overwhelmed, spent, anxious, lonely, guilty, unappreciated, ashamed, angry, reactive, scared, discouraged, frustrated, or sad. When we are hurt by the lack of gratitude or support from our family and exhausted by our invisible load. When we give our absolute best, yet we see no progress or rewards. When we wonder where we went wrong or if we've gotten it all wrong. When the constant influx of needs and demands keeps us living in survival mode. When we try to be strong for everyone, yet inside we just want to scream.

And it is that dichotomy—where we look strong and capable externally, yet feel mounting tension internally—that drives a mom to her breaking point. Even mothers who hit all the marks may not be well or on a good path. For this reason, we need to talk about a mom's inner life. We need safe places to process our struggles and needs, friends who listen and empathize, and healthy conversations that move us forward so we can genuinely thrive.

My friend, this book is designed to serve that purpose. I hope to be the friend to you that my friends have been to me. I may not know your journey (whether you have one child or seven, boys or girls, toddlers or teenagers, babies you birthed or children you adopted), but I can assume this:

*You love your family passionately. Yet the same love that **drives** you can also **deplete** you because it never feels like enough.*

With motherhood, there is no stopping point. There is no clocking out, checking out, or leaving work behind. As your kids grow up, the demands on you multiply. Boundaries blur, life gets real, and you get stretched too thin.

Mothers sacrifice (it is what we do best), yet sometimes in our determination to love our people well, we overextend ourselves. We can get lost in our support roles, tending to everyone else's needs while forgetting about our own. We prioritize the wellness of our loved ones at the expense of our wellness. *We let sacrifices evolve into quiet self-neglect.*

> *We take our sick children to the doctor—yet push*
> *through our illnesses.*
> *We bathe our baby every day—yet skip our own*
> *shower.*
> *We enforce our toddler's bedtime—yet stay up until*
> *2:00 a.m. to finish our work.*
> *We sign up our five-year-old for soccer and tennis—yet*
> *don't consider a personal hobby.*
> *We make our kids sit down and eat whole meals—yet*
> *eat protein bars on the run.*
> *We seek therapy for our struggling teen—yet wrestle*
> *with our problems alone.*
> *We give our family a soft place to land—yet shoulder*
> *the burden of everyone's pain, even if it crushes us,*
> *to keep a happy, peaceful home.*

In short, we dismiss our own needs to serve as Givers. We carry on long after our minds, bodies, and spirits tell us to rest or quit. We forget that we are, first and foremost, human beings. We hold unrealistic expectations of what it means to be human.

We wonder why we hit brick walls, see the wheels fall off, and beg someone to throw us a bone because we are *exhausted*.

In your journey as a Giver, you work overtime. You try hard to be the best mom, person, and role model you can be. You're scared to fail because the stakes are high, yet even on good days, you may feel like you are failing someone. You have a critic in your head who picks you (and your choices) apart.

What if I told you 1) you're doing better than you think, 2) your kids aren't critiquing you the way you critique yourself, 3) you have value and purpose beyond your role as a mom, and 4) to serve your family well, you must tend to your needs and wellness too?

After all, you can only take your children as far as you have come. Raising healthy kids begins with them seeing a healthy mom. If you're not in a healthy place (or working to get there), then failure on your part is more likely. You'll struggle to find the strength, stamina, patience, and presence you need to be a healthy Giver.

In their book *The Power of Showing Up*, *New York Times* bestselling authors Dr. Daniel Siegel and Dr. Tina Payne Bryson say children need four things for healthy development: they need to feel safe, seen, soothed, and secure. Parents who show up and offer a quality of presence help their children thrive.[2]

Dr. Bryson says, "One of the very best scientific predictors for how any child turns out—in terms of happiness, social skills, mental health, academic success, and meaningful relationships—is whether at least one adult in their life has consistently shown up for them."[3] These findings, based on brain and attachment research, remind us of how important it is to simply engage with our children, pay attention to their lives, and be emotionally stable and available.

Motherhood motivates, and knowing that your health

directly impacts your children is a powerful incentive. With that in mind, I wrote this book. *It's your guide to inner wellness and includes ten ways to grow stronger from the inside out through ten life habits you can incorporate to become the mother, woman, and role model you are meant to be.*

The best part is you don't have to be perfect. Why? Because perfect parents don't prepare their children for an imperfect world. Perfect parents don't admit their need for Jesus or acknowledge their own struggles. The older your children get, the more you parent with *influence* rather than *power*. Instead of seeing your trials as defeats, see the opportunities. When you respond in healthy ways, you prepare your children for their trials. You give them a model to draw on during their own dark days.

This reference point matters because your children mostly see perfection (perceived, not real). They scroll through social media and think something must be wrong with them since everyone else is living the dream. Even well-meaning parents can feed this illusion, and I often think about the seventeen-year-old girl who cried to her parents during a heart-to-heart talk as she finally admitted, "You two are just so perfect, and I feel like I can never measure up!"

Her parents were heartbroken because they never intended to portray that image. Yet sometimes, in our effort to be good role models, we hide our humanity. While we certainly shouldn't burden our children with problems best taken to other adults, it does help them to see us cope with some problems in positive, productive ways.

None of us imagined, as we cradled newborn babies, that one day we'd have to parent while also handling Major League stress. We didn't realize how much strength and resilience we'd need to handle the heartaches life can bring.

Your journey as a mother may get lonely, but you are never

alone. You always have Jesus and the Holy Spirit (God's presence in the heart of believers) to strengthen, empower, and guide you. In John 16:33 (NIV) Jesus says, "I have told you these things, so that in me you may have peace. In this world you will have trouble. But take heart! I have overcome the world." Without Jesus, you are powerless, but with Him you grow equipped. You have God's mighty power on your side.

As moms, we often need permission to take better care of ourselves. We long to reach our full potential without vanity, guilt, or obsession. Your greatest life purpose, even greater than motherhood, is to know, love, and serve God. As you journey toward genuine wellness, you also journey toward Him. You become a light for those who know you.

Wellness helps you become the best version of yourself so you can bravely and boldly serve God. It makes you a good steward of the gifts He has given you, such as your family, your body, your soul, and your time. Even exceptional Givers have legitimate needs as humans, and as you read on, I pray you feel loved by the ultimate Giver, who sacrificed His only Son for you and restores you when you grow weary.

> Every good and perfect gift is from above, coming down from the Father of the heavenly lights, who does not change like shifting shadows.
>
> JAMES 1:17 (NIV)

INSPIRE YOUR KIDS TO OUTDO YOU

A panel of moms raising teenagers spoke to young moms. Their main takeaway was this:

*Don't run yourself so hard during the day
that you have nothing left to give when
your kids come home from school.*

Wow, this speaks to me. Too often, the reason why I feel depleted is because I've worked myself to my limits. It only takes one rude comment from a child or one email with an urgent deadline to push me over the edge.

The good news is, I know myself. I'm aware of what works (and doesn't work) in my life. I also know, as the mom of three teenagers and one preteen, that older kids have keen observational skills. My children will always remember what they witness in my life right now, and as I prepare them for the real world, I focus on two things: their health and their relationship with God.

Ultimately, these things matter most, and if they get them right, their lives will fall into order.

This is equally true for you. You may be quick to sacrifice, but don't sacrifice your wellness. Don't forget the hidden benefits of modeling a healthy adult lifestyle. By doing this well, you give your children a head start. *You equip them to outdo you.*

And isn't that the goal of parenting? Don't we all want our kids to outdo us, to live lives that are longer, smarter, and more fruitful than the lives we have lived?

My dad once counseled a college boy who got upset over his little brother's athletic talent. Beginning in middle school, this little brother exceeded his big brother's records. My father told the elder son, "You better *hope* your little brother does better than you, because that means you did your job!"

In short, it is our job to turn around and empower those behind us. We are called to help them, inspire them, and set a good example. Your life gains purpose as you allow the next generation to learn from your mistakes and build on what you started. Let them see a picture of wellness, and watch them carry that knowledge with them as they get launched into the future.

> Like arrows in the hands of a warrior are children born in one's youth.
>
> PSALM 127:4 (NIV)

JOIN THIS JOURNEY

This book will release just before my fiftieth birthday. At this point, I'm reflecting on the past, dreaming about the future, and aiming to stay healthy and strong for the second half of my life.

Rarely does a mother's strength look like the cover of a fitness magazine. More often, it plays out in subtle ways. It may look like

- showing your vulnerable side
- admitting you need help
- begging God to heal your child
- holding it together as you watch your child suffer
- insisting on answers to a mystery illness
- attending a party alone
- mustering the courage to make new friends
- starting over
- moving back in with your parents
- finding a job
- advocating for your child
- watching your son choose his wife and get married
- letting your daughter pull away and become independent
- ending a toxic relationship
- standing alone in a decision
- parenting a disagreeable teenager
- selling prized possessions to afford professional help for your child

- being kind to an unkind person
- parenting a child who requires extra love and attention
- building a relationship with a difficult child
- listening to hard truths
- persevering in prayer
- fighting temptation
- apologizing
- forgiving
- showing yourself compassion and grace
- feeling your feelings
- breaking a destructive cycle
- biting your tongue
- controlling your temper
- saying good-bye to your parents
- saying good-bye to your child leaving home
- taking a baby step only God can see.

When I was a young girl, I couldn't understand why my mom cried over laundry or because she felt tired. I thought her life purpose was to serve me, and I cringe when I think about all the times that I acted ungrateful, shrugged her off, or dumped on her as an easy target.

I owe my mom many apologies, and only now do I realize that she had more love and inner strength than I ever gave her credit for. Only now can I see her as the Giver she was.

I can't undo the past, but I can honor my mom's legacy by encouraging you. I can remind you that your children may be so wrapped up in their lives that they forget about your needs, so if you don't address your needs, who will?

Motherhood is deeply rewarding, but most moms are underappreciated. It may take years (or decades) for our children to see us through a mature lens, and, in the meantime, we need each other. We need uplifting voices in the trenches. After all, it takes a Giver to "get" a Giver and value the work she does.

So, gather your most trusted friends to study this book with you. Start meaningful conversations with like-minded moms who bolster and celebrate women.

Even if your children are your greatest game-changer, you are more than just their mom. You have a place in this world beyond serving them. Your secret weapon as they grow up, the way you parent them from a distance, is through your influence. Believe it or not, some of your best parenting will come through the example you set and the determination you model as you learn to value yourself and your life.

Now, join me on this journey to wellness that will expand your faith, your relationships, and your perspective of yourself.

Do not despise these small beginnings, for the LORD rejoices
to see the work begin . . .

ZECHARIAH 4:10 (NLT)

REFLECTION QUESTIONS

1. How high of a priority is your wellness to you? Have you ever paid the price for neglecting it?

2. How has motherhood changed you? What has surprised you in the best and worst ways?

3. Name three things you do for your children that you should (but don't) do for yourself.

4. Some parents try to replicate their childhood. Others hope to do it different and better. Where do you fall?

What past experiences have impacted the way you balance your family's needs with your own?

5. What does strength look like in your life right now? How has that picture changed from five years ago?

6. Think of a healthy Giver you know. What habits do they practice?

KNOW YOUR WORTH

A Mother Needs to Feel Valued

*Your value doesn't decrease based on
someone's inability to see your worth.*

ANONYMOUS

The pediatrician made friendly conversation with my fourteen-year-old daughter as she scanned her body at her annual checkup.

They laughed as they talked about Halloween costumes and making slime at home.

As the pediatrician finished, she sat down in her rolling chair. She smiled at my daughter, the same age as her daughter, and leaned in. I'd been to enough visits to know that this was where she switched gears from doctor mode to mom mode. She'd focus less on my daughter's body and more on my daughter's heart.

"As a teenager," the pediatrician explained, "you'll have a lot of new experiences in the years ahead. Boys will enter the picture, and some won't be that great. I want you to always remember something."

The doctor leaned in and paused for emphasis. "Always remember that *you* are a *gift*. Some people won't treat you like a gift, but that doesn't change your value. You are still a gift no matter what anyone else says or thinks. You got that?"

My daughter nodded, not fully understanding the context. I blinked back tears because I did understand, and I was thankful for this truth being impressed on her heart.

In this new season, my daughter and her friends would get a taste of adulthood. They'd meet people who are quick to use or manipulate others. Some encounters would make them feel rejected, insignificant, disposable, or overlooked. Inevitably, they'd question their worth. They'd wonder what must be wrong with them to make a guy (or a girl) act in hurtful ways.

Before these realities kicked in, our pediatrician wanted my daughter to know her value. *Because when you know that you are a gift, you don't let hurtful people define you.* You protect the gifts God gives you, like your confidence and self-esteem.

It pained me to imagine anyone treating my baby as less than a gift. Yet I knew it was only a matter of time before someone would come along and try.

I often think of this story when I see women struggle with self-worth. I've struggled myself, and chances are, you have too.

Why? Because one irony of the sexes is that while men tend to struggle with *pride,* women tend to struggle with *insecurity.* While males tend to think too much of themselves, females tend to think too little of themselves. Our culture of "girl power" tries to counter this, but this confidence often takes a narcissistic view of self. It's about self-worship, not self-love, and confidence like that isn't healthy or sustainable.

My pediatrician's advice to my daughter is equally true for you. No matter where you've been or what you've been through in the past, *you* are a *gift.* That truth still stands regardless of old wounds and hurts. *Your value comes from within because you were born with inherent dignity.* And if you could see yourself the way God looks at you, with the loving gaze of a proud Father, you'd never question your worth again.

What God creates, God loves, and what God loves, He loves forever. Even on your worst days, He loves you at maximum capacity. Love begins with God because God *is* love. He doesn't love us because we are good; He loves us because He is good. Thankfully, His love doesn't depend on what any human being does or says.

God loves you first, and He invites you to respond to His love. Open your heart to receive His transforming grace. Embrace Jesus as your Savior, and unlock the gift of the Holy Spirit. As

God's grace works inside of you, it empowers you to love yourself (and others) in response to what Jesus did on the cross.

> Whoever does not love does not know God, because God is love. This is how God showed his love among us: He sent his one and only Son into the world that we might live through him. This is love: not that we loved God, but that he loved us and sent his Son as an atoning sacrifice for our sins.
>
> 1 JOHN 4:8–10 (NIV)

WORSHIP THE RIGHT GOD

I'm sure you have had days when you loved your people, yet your people didn't love you back.

It hurts, doesn't it? Whether it is your child, your spouse, a family member, or a friend, feeling your love go unreciprocated is a dagger in the heart.

When this happens to me, I try to remember that we, as humans, are sinful. We hurt the people we love sometimes because we're in a mood, going through a phase, wrestling with a problem, or feeling some brokenness that impacts our behavior.

I love my people with all my heart, but relying on them to always make me feel worthy sets the stage for disappointment. It keeps my confidence at the mercy of their fickle human nature.

Like me, they are a work in progress. They have baggage, backstories, and blind spots. If I measure my worth based on how they treat me today or whether they reciprocate my efforts, then I'm in for a rocky ride. I've rooted my faith in the wrong thing, elevating people over God and putting people on a pedestal they're not meant to live on.

The truth is, people make terrible gods. *And even the biggest blessings stop being blessings when you make them the center of your universe.*

God created us to worship Him, and if we don't put Him first, we'll find substitutes. We'll worship false idols like our family, our friends, our body, our job, our image, our money, our accomplishments, or some earthly trapping.

Dr. Tim Keller says, "You don't get to decide to worship. Everyone worships something. The only choice you get is what to worship."[1] We all get our priorities out of whack. We've all based our worth on something other than God and rooted our identity in something other than Christ.

Recently a mom emailed me after her son cheated on a test. She was heartbroken for obvious reasons—and because this cheating was out of character. As moms do, she blamed herself. She felt like she had failed her son and saw this decision as a reflection of her parenting.

So often we base our value on our loved ones' decisions or our relationship with them. *We gauge our self-worth based on results and absorb their failures as our failures.* Of the many hats we wear, of the many support roles we play, our roles as moms feel most significant and high stakes.

To no surprise, motherhood is the most common platform on which we build our identity. When our children thrive, we feel great, and when they fail, we blame ourselves. We grieve and wonder where we went wrong.

It is undeniably true that we, as parents, influence our children's choices. It is also true that our children choose their own path. They're separate from us, and they have free will. The older they get, the less control we have, and even if we could parent perfectly, we're not guaranteed results. Even Jesus, a perfect role model, had one disciple betray Him. Judas knew better, yet he went against everything that Jesus had taught him.

Thankfully, your worth doesn't depend on the choices your children make or how well they perform. It isn't tied to how desirable you are to your spouse, how many girls' trips you get invited to, how popular you are, what you weigh, whether you can rock a bikini, how productive you've been lately, your Instagram likes, your salary, how many people you please, what your mother-in-law thinks of you, or what your ex-husband spews in a text.

Your core identity—the one that runs deeper than your identity as a mother, wife, sister, friend, daughter, colleague, boss, etc.—is that you are a child of God. He invites you into His family through the saving grace of Christ. When you accept this invitation, God works in you and through you by the power of the Holy Spirit. The same spirit that raised Jesus from the dead is what God gives to those who believe in Christ.

You are worthy because God made you. He created you in His image and for a unique purpose. Nothing about you is a mistake because God doesn't make mistakes. And when you base your identity on Christ and the sacrifice He made, you build your self-worth on a solid foundation. You gain a confidence that lasts because it is rooted in eternal life, not circumstances that may change overnight.

My friend Shannon had an epiphany during a pilgrimage to the Holy Land. While praying in the garden of Gethsemane, she heard Jesus tell her, "I didn't die to make you worthy. I died because you *are* worthy." These words settled Shannon's doubt about her inherent value. Jesus died for her, and now she lives for Him.

A. W. Tozer said, "As God is exalted to the right place in our lives, a thousand problems are solved all at once."[2] Making God your number-one priority brings clarity and strength. It sets the stage for right-ordered living. It reduces the urge to worship people or chase after human approval. It keeps false idols off the pedestal and allows you to build a strong identity.

The secret to knowing your worth is to embrace God's love for you. Even when you don't like yourself, even when your life is a wreck, you are priceless to Him. Trust eternal truths, not short-lived opinions, when deciding what to believe. Your value comes from within, and as you unlock this mystery, it draws your heart closer to Him.

> And I am convinced that nothing can ever separate us from God's love. Neither death nor life, neither angels nor demons, neither our fears for today nor our worries about tomorrow— not even the powers of hell can separate us from God's love.
>
> ROMANS 8:38 (NLT)

EMBRACE HEALTHY SELF-LOVE

In recent years, *self-love* and *self-care* have become major buzz words.

For some people, they've gained a negative connotation as they get used to justify an excessive focus on self. Under the guise of *self-love* or *self-care,* we can make excuses for any lifestyle or habit: from exercising three hours a day, to taking monthly vacations, to overindulging in life's pleasures, to leaving our family or quitting our life because they no longer make us happy.

Practically anything counts as self-love these days, and when we exceed the limits of reason or moderation, we become a narcissistic culture fixated on self-gratification. We buy or pursue anything that makes us feel better, yet still leaves us empty because our pursuits are all about us.

We aren't meant to live this way. And one reason why

Americans feel so lonely is because our culture of self-reliance, autonomy, and excessive self-focus disconnects us. It is hard to find community or real friends when we only look out for ourselves.

At the other extreme are people who neglect themselves. They work their fingers to the bone, pouring out yet never refilling, giving to the point of depletion. In many cases, they undervalue themselves. They let people drain them. They believe they are worth less than the average person and often feel powerless over their lives.

Neither extreme is healthy. *Both self-worship and self-neglect are destructive and prevent us from reaching our full potential and serving our God-given purpose.*

So how do you get yourself (and keep yourself) in a healthy place? How can you practice self-love and self-care in a way that brings life?

The starting point is God. And the best explanation I've seen comes from the book *Boundaries*. The authors, Dr. Henry Cloud and Dr. John Townsend, explain how God gives you your *life*, your *time*, and your *body* as gifts, and it is your responsibility to protect your gifts. You are called to be a good steward of your gifts by setting mental, physical, emotional, and spiritual boundaries that distinguish what is and isn't your responsibility.

Many women struggle to set boundaries. They care deeply about their relationships and let people cross lines or pile their burdens on them because they're scared of what may happen if they show a backbone. The authors of *Boundaries* write:

> There are two reasons why you need others to help with boundaries. The first is that *your most basic need in life is for relationship.* People suffer much to have relationships, and many put up with abuse because they fear their partners will leave them and they will be alone if they stand up to them.

Fear of being alone keeps many in hurtful patterns for years. They are afraid that if they set boundaries they will not have any love in their life.[3]

I have a friend who is editing a book for a man who grew up in poverty. He has a great testimony, and his come-to-Jesus moment occurred when he got two girls pregnant in quick succession. In sharing about his childhood, he says his mom was adamant in teaching him and his brothers to respect women. When it came to her own life, however, she didn't make men respect her. She endured more than she should have because she didn't know her worth.

I also have a friend whose husband is in law enforcement. She recently told me about Badge Bunnies, women who pursue and sleep with police officers, often getting passed around. It used to make her mad and judgmental, but now that she is older, it makes her sad. She understands how there must be a deep or hidden pain to make Badge Bunnies devalue themselves.

Stories like this break my heart, and they also explain why we should talk about healthy self-love, because far too many women don't value or respect themselves.

The fact is, you matter. *Your life isn't an accident, because God created you for a purpose, to serve your generation like no one in the universe has ever served before.* I know this is hard to believe when your days feel mundane, when your biggest feat is folding laundry, cleaning the bathroom toilets, or deodorizing your son's athletic bag, but it is true.

Even if you've taken wrong turns, made big mistakes, or been told that you're a worthless burden, God can use you in powerful ways. He can help you see yourself and others through new eyes.

This is pivotal because it distinguishes truth from lies. Chances are, you have met some liars before, and you understand how one flippant remark, such as, "You'll never amount to anything!" or "You're nothing without me!" can leave a lasting scar. It can mess with your psyche, shatter your self-image, and become the core message of your identity.

Of all the liars you have met, the most dangerous one is the critic in your head. It makes toxic statements such as

- It's too late.
- You're no longer needed.
- You've ruined everything.
- You don't belong.
- Nobody likes you. Quit trying to make friends.
- You're a terrible person and a horrible mom.
- You can't handle this.
- Your life doesn't matter.
- You'll never recover.
- You don't deserve food. You're fat enough already.
- Are you kidding? Look at yourself! You're a joke.
- You're no fun anymore. Your glory days are behind you.
- You don't deserve a good life or a good guy. Get over it.
- Your mom/dad/crazy ex was right—you're worthless. Something is wrong with you.

The problem with these statements is 1) they keep you stuck, 2) they twist the truth, and 3) they're not from God. God created you to live with a spirit of strength, not defeat. He speaks the truth in love, not condemnation. He wants you to live a healthy, vibrant life where you rely on Him for all your needs.

Self-loathing isn't from God, and neither is shame. Shame convinces you to struggle alone and let no one in to help. It points you toward isolation where no one can speak truth or counter the lies in your head. It tells you there is no hope.

Dr. Brené Brown says empathy is the antidote to shame. "If you put shame in a Petri dish," she explains, "it needs three things to grow exponentially: secrecy, silence, and judgment. If you put the same amount of shame in a Petri dish and douse it with empathy, it can't survive. The two most powerful words when we're in a struggle: me too."[4]

So how do you find empathy? Through compassionate people. People who see the real you and love you despite your flaws. People who are self-aware and admit their own failures and shortcomings. People who generously give grace and understand the healing power of Jesus. People who want what is best for you and won't let you settle for less.

Empathetic people build real community. They offer a safe place to work through your struggles or shame. You aren't meant to do life alone, and though I'll dive deeper into community in the friendship chapter, it is worth mentioning now that spending time with people who love you helps you better love yourself. *When someone knows your unvarnished truths and still considers you amazing, you get a glimpse of God's love.*

In Romans 7:15 (NIV) Paul wrote, "I do not understand what I do. For what I want to do I do not do, but what I hate I do." Who can't relate to Paul's honesty? Who hasn't felt the pain of doing what we *know* we shouldn't do and then hating ourselves for it?

Self-love requires truth-telling. It means pulling back the curtain to do a fearless self-inventory of your sins (in Greek, the word *sin* means "to miss the mark," the benchmark set by Jesus) and to do better moving forward. God knows you aren't perfect, and that's why His mercy is greater than any mistake imaginable. Once you confess your sins, He forgets them so you can live in the freedom of Christ (Isaiah 43:25).

Being honest with yourself (about who you've been, who you are, and who you hope to be) connects your past to your future. God loves you unconditionally, and having that security enables you to examine your life and identify what holds you back.

What temptations trip you up? What situations make you weak? What habits wreak havoc? How can you work toward health and positive goals? What keeps you from becoming the best version of yourself? What uncomfortable truth should come to light?

> *Maybe you're exhausted because you overcommit and can't say "no."*
>
> *Maybe you wrestle with jealousy and comparison as you see the blessings that others enjoy.*
>
> *Maybe you're stressed because you feel responsible for making everyone happy, and their emotions weigh you down.*
>
> *Maybe you settle for bad relationships because you desperately want to be loved and can't break the cycle.*
>
> *Maybe you drink to excess because nobody taught you how to cope. You'd rather numb your emotions than feel them.*
>
> *Maybe you struggle to show love because nobody loved you. It is a challenge, even with your family.*
>
> *Maybe you feel overwhelmed because you never learned to identify and navigate your emotions, much less your child's emotions.*
>
> *Maybe your breakdowns are rooted in trauma from the past.*

*Maybe you hustle because achievements earn you
   praise.*
*Maybe you put up with mean friends because they're
   social and fun.*
*Maybe you gossip to feel better in comparison or to
   connect with a gossipy friend.*
*Maybe you refuse to rest because productivity fuels
   your sense of worth.*
*Maybe you feel powerless, bitter, or always wronged
   because you live life as a victim.*
*Maybe you're unhappy with your kids or spouse
   because they aren't what you dreamed of.*
*Maybe you're angry because you've repressed your hard
   emotions.*
*Maybe you feel empty because you've neglected your
   soul and inner growth.*

**Feeling insecure and unworthy will make you act in inse-
cure and unworthy ways.** Feeling stuck will make you live
defeated. God created you for more, and though He loves you
exactly as you are today, He loves you too much to leave you
there. He has bigger plans for your future, plans to reveal your
untapped potential.

You can't lose God's love, even if you don't love yourself. Even
if you reject Him or run away, He'll pursue you. Like the shep-
herd in Matthew 18:12 who leaves ninety-nine sheep to search
for the one sheep that is lost, God would travel to the ends of the
earth for you. You're not just another face in the crowd. To Him,
you're fully seen, desired, and known.

**God knew at the beginning of time that our world would
need you for this moment in time.** Self-love evolves as you

deepen your relationship with Him, let Him love you, and embrace your purpose. You are a gift, and though some people won't treat you as a gift, they can't change God's mind. He knows the truth—that your value is rooted in Him—and He planted that truth in your heart before the day you were born.

> For you formed my inward parts; you knitted me together in my mother's womb. I praise you, for I am fearfully and wonderfully made. Wonderful are your works; my soul knows it very well.
>
> PSALM 139:13–14 (ESV)

What Knowing Your Worth Models for Your Child

When my husband told me that his job required a move to Houston, I was devastated. I'd lived in Birmingham for most of my adult life, and I'd built an amazing community for myself and my children.

My friends were my lifeline. Together we had survived newborns and toddlers and built a nice economy of play dates and carpools. I loved my book club, my supper club, my birthday club, and all the monthly gatherings where we shared inside jokes and old stories. I dreamed of us growing old together and playing bridge at eighty years old!

Uprooting this dream rocked my world, and for weeks I cried in my pillow. Moving to a huge international city was daunting, and helping three children re-create their lives (two in the throes of middle school) felt overwhelming. Normal securities were replaced by giant uncertainties.

In Houston, I got lost and needed my GPS every time I left our driveway. Internally, I felt lost too, unmoored without my friends and exhausted since being a newcomer felt like an ongoing job interview.

As my insecurities grew, I asked God to keep them from seeping into our lives. Things that would not have fazed me in Birmingham became major hurdles. My youngest son, for instance, asked to try baseball. I knew his Houston friends had been playing for years and were far better than him. Before I even signed him up, I dreaded the thought of him standing alone at bat. I was afraid that he might embarrass himself (and me).

My husband, who moved often growing up, offered perspective and stability. He reminded me how our children would move repeatedly in life, but the One they worship would never change. We chose our church before our home and let God's love for us be our anchor.

Today, I see God's provision. He has answered our prayers for friendship, strengthened my marriage, and recentered my identity in Christ as I let go of the idol of "being known." While I still need my GPS to find the grocery store, internally I'm not so lost. I trust God's plan and see His hand in the details, like when my son scored a run in baseball. Ultimately, God is our only guarantee, and as I've learned myself, I pray my children realize that He is enough.

Kristin Denson Sartelle
mom of two sons and one daughter

REFLECTION QUESTIONS

1. Name a time when you doubted your worth. Did a person, event, or remark trigger it? Did you work through the doubt or let it redefine you? Explain.

2. Name an idol you put before God. When it fails or disappoints you, what is the lesson?

3. Name toxic statements made by the critic in your head. What truths counter these lies?

4. Do you believe God loves you and that you can't lose His love? Why or why not?

5. What does healthy self-love and self-care look like to you?

6. What situations or life changes have triggered your insecurity? Moving forward, how can you mentally prepare for insecure moments?

2

REST

A Mother Needs to Feel Restored

*Listen, are you breathing just a
little, and calling it a life?*

Mary Oliver[1]

One morning in January, I met some moms for coffee and listened as one mom shared a story from the Christmas holidays.

On a busy Saturday, as she ran circles around the house trying to decorate and tackle her to-do list, her husband kicked back in the den to watch college football.

Each time that she passed him, her irritation rose. With a drink in one hand and a crackling fire at his feet, her husband looked annoyingly at peace.

He was so relaxed, in fact, that he didn't notice how busy she was, much less offer to help.

Inside her, another fire started. After her third or fourth trip, she stopped moving and lit into her husband, telling him, "Quit enjoying yourself!"

Every mom having coffee that day laughed out loud and nodded. We practically high-fived her, as if to say, "We get it, sister, we've been there too!" This scenario could have played out in any of our homes and, chances are, you can relate.

In many homes, this is a common dynamic. *Where we live is also where we do most of our work as mothers, and from an empty fridge to a leaky faucet to a room that needs Christmas magic, something always calls for our attention.*

Most of us don't aspire to be Pinterest moms because we're perfectly content to be Amazon Prime moms. But, as my father says, our parenting years are also our working years, and that requires a major juggling act. Even if we dial back and lower expectations, we still stay busy. We're still managing carpools, calendars, meals, needs, emotions, problems, deadlines, home maintenance, appointments, aging parents, and a host of other responsibilities.

Throw in a sick child or a sudden crisis, and you may feel stretched so thin that you snap.

In my younger days, I didn't believe in rest. Especially as a new mom, full of adrenaline and caffeine, my reserve didn't feel empty because my heart felt so full. When I was tired, a nap made everything better. I was good to go again.

But with age I have changed my tune. I have seen firsthand how not making time for rest leads to burnout, exhaustion, loneliness, emptiness, and lost joy. Some exhaustion can't be cured with a nap, a vacation, or traditional ideas of self-care. *Some exhaustion seeps deeply into our bones, and only time with God and healthy lifestyle rhythms can truly restore us.*

Sadly, we often feel like we can't rest as moms. We worry that if we stop moving, we may crash or lose momentum.

And what then? Who will hold the family together? What if it all comes unglued? What if our rest leads to chaos and we end up more stressed than before? The mothership can't go down!

Nobody knows the family juggling act like a mom, so we stay in motion and resign ourselves to living with overwhelm.

Clearly, this isn't sustainable. And when we stay in this cycle, our family begins to feel like a burden. We get irritated when they enjoy themselves as we work hard. We become the resentful moms that we swore we would never be. We look at old pictures from our teenage years and wonder what ever happened to that happy, carefree girl.

She is still there, ready to enjoy life again, but right now she may be buried beneath the demands of motherhood. She may need a way out and permission to just *be*.

Believe it or not, the world will keep turning if you rest. Your family won't go up in flames, and you won't lose momentum.

Instead, you'll recharge. You'll gain some distance from your stress and later laugh as you share stories over coffee. You'll feel lighter as you bond with other moms over the highs and lows of life.

In the Bible, Jesus talked about rest and giving our burdens to Him. He modeled healthy lifestyle rhythms by taking spiritual, physical, and mental breaks. Since people always needed Him, He set boundaries around His time. He showed us how to rest, even in times of pressure.

- Before choosing the twelve apostles, Jesus retreated to a mountaintop to pray all night. (Luke 6:12–13)
- In the middle of a fierce storm with His disciples, He fell asleep on a boat. (Matthew 8:24)
- After hearing about John the Baptist's death, He withdrew on a boat to grieve in a solitary place. (Matthew 14:13)
- He ate His last meal before death with only His disciples. (Matthew 26:17–29)
- He kept the Sabbath holy. (Luke 4:16)

Two sisters named Mary and Martha had opposite responses when Jesus visited. While Martha, the practical and efficient sister, busily prepared for the Lord, Mary just wanted to sit at His feet. Martha resented her sister for not working. She asked Jesus to tell Mary to help her.

Jesus said, "Martha, Martha . . . you are worried and upset about many things, but few things are needed—or indeed only one. Mary has chosen what is better, and it will not be taken away from her" (Luke 10:41–42, NIV).

Rest is essential to everyone's health. It recalibrates the soul, amplifies God's voice, and helps us find peace at the feet of Jesus.

Next to His enormous love, everything else feels small. Worries, demands, and fears shrink into their rightful place.

Rest has never felt more elusive because we live in a world of unrest. Besides your family and personal responsibilities, you face twenty-four/seven demands for your time—nonstop emails, beeps, and notifications—that make everything feel urgent.

It is not all urgent, and with God's help you can prioritize what is *important* over what is *urgent*. You can set healthy boundaries that prevent interruptions from bleeding into your life. What someone else considers "urgent" may not be part of God's plan for you, and rather than let outside demands drive your schedule, you can make time to retreat and listen to Him.

Life is too short to live with your hair on fire. You are too loved by God to never take a break. You are a human *being*, not a human *doing*, and while there is certainly a time to work, there is also a time to stop, breathe, pray, and give thanks for your life.

"Be still, and know that I am God! I will be honored by every nation. I will be honored throughout the world."

PSALM 46:10 (NLT)

PACE YOURSELF

When I was in college, the band Alabama released a song called "I'm in a Hurry to Get Things Done." The lyrics talk about rushing around until life is no fun, and with my Type-A personality, I felt as if they were written for me. Even now when I hear this song, I feel called out and reminded to slow down, chill, and enjoy the present moment.

The truth is, relaxing can be hard for me, especially when there is work to do. I've heard it said that humans tend to veer toward **burnout** or **inaction,** and when you're a naturally driven person who thrives on activity, burnout is the common path. While part of me wishes I wasn't this way, I also know that God designed me this way and I'm not alone.

Many people have trouble with rest. In fact, there is evidence of a cultural problem based on the many bestselling products and trends that promise to ease our stress. Things like weighted blankets, CBD oil, essential oils, melatonin tablets, diffusers, therapy dogs, sound machines, yoga, meditation, aromatherapy candles, silent retreats, and popular apps like Headspace and Calm are all signs of our times. They reveal how desperate we are to escape the frantic pace of society and the restlessness inside our minds.

Why is rest so difficult? And why do we feel guilty about adding breathing room to our schedules? Because in countries like America, we glorify the hustle. We praise overachievers (and achievements) and treat busy like a badge of honor. We brag about running on four hours of sleep. We are expected to always be "on" and available through technology.

When I was growing up, it was considered rude to call someone after 9:00 p.m. Families had a buffer that let them rejuvenate at home. But now, that buffer is gone. It is no longer taboo to reach out at a crazy hour. Today's world has no boundaries, and this puts more demands on your time. It gives you more ways to spend your time and compare yourself to other moms.

If you're a go-getter, a people-pleaser, an extrovert, or a Type-A personality like me, you may find it particularly hard to resist the urge to always respond quickly. You may keep up an impossible pace because you like to feel accomplished and stay in the good graces of others.

But when activity is your comfort zone, when staying busy helps you self-soothe, when you don't have time to sit with your thoughts, pray, or reflect, then you start to lose yourself. *Rest feels awkward, peace becomes elusive, and you miss the signs that God sends your way.*

This past autumn, I missed a stunning tree with changing leaves in my neighbor's yard. My youngest daughter raved about it as I drove her to school one morning, and she told me to view it from my bedroom porch. She said it was red and amazing, and I had to see it! I intended to do it, but I forgot. A week later, she told me that all the leaves had fallen. I'd missed my chance to witness this gift outside my bedroom window. Apparently, nature doesn't wait until my to-do list is done.

We all have work to do, and we all want our lives to matter. But we'll never be our best selves or reach our goals if we constantly fire on all cylinders and work at a breakneck speed. To go the distance, we must pace ourselves. We need grace and downtime.

If you're in a season where you feel tapped out, it's okay. Jesus can work with a small offering and cares most about the heart behind it. He turned two fish and five loaves of bread from a young boy into a feast for 5,000 people (John 6:1-14). He lived a quiet life until he was thirty and had a ministry that lasted only three years—yet look at Christianity's impact still today.

Even when you are limited, God is unlimited. Even when you rest and heal, He works behind the scenes. He loves you always, regardless of what you bring to the table, and He wants you to take time to replenish your soul.

> Why, you do not even know what will happen tomorrow. What is your life? You are a mist that appears for a little while and then vanishes.
>
> JAMES 4:14 (NIV)

MOTHER YOURSELF

Many of us learn the hard way why rest matters.

It often takes a mental breakdown, a physical breakdown, or a health crisis to open our eyes and force changes in how we manage our lives.

A very active and athletic mom suddenly faced an injury that kept her down for six weeks. She told her friends, "God gave me a speeding ticket." Her downtime helped her see the distractions in her busy life. She was glad for the intervention that forced her to slow down.

In my own life, I've learned that as we age, we must "mother" ourselves because eventually we all will lose the generation that raised us. Our mothers can no longer nag us and, surprisingly, since losing my mother a few years ago, I miss that. I miss my mom looking out for my well-being like nobody else on the planet. Since no one can fill her shoes, the responsibility is now mine.

So how do you mother yourself? By taking care of yourself mentally, physically, emotionally, and spiritually. By paying close attention and tending to your needs. By checking in with yourself regularly—and seeking help or making changes when you aren't well.

You also mother yourself by not stretching yourself too thin. Creating space in your calendar creates space in your head. Both play a role in your ability to rest.

Following are some ways to enable space, rest, and peace in your life.

Set Boundaries.

Boundaries draw a line between what is yours to carry—and what is not. They protect your soul, your sanity, your sleep, and your time. If you don't set boundaries, people will drain you. You'll do things that you don't want to do and aren't called to do.

A friend said this:

> I always felt I had to be there for everybody at the exact moment people needed me (stop and drop for friends and family). As I entered my late forties, I felt overwhelmed. I didn't have the energy I once had, yet I kept trying to keep the pace and be present for everybody. It became a struggle.
>
> *Who am I? What is my purpose?* I had let people drain me to the point that I didn't know who I was anymore or what I was supposed to be doing. Age has taught me my limitations and tolerance levels, who to let in and who to keep out. That has given me strength and helped me to grow. I've learned to speak my truth and not feel guilty for saying *no* or for stating why I've said *no.* It is through learning my weaknesses that I gained the strength to be stronger and help others.

Many women struggle to set boundaries because they're afraid to make people unhappy or mad. They get their worth from external approval, and after years of bending over backward to accommodate others, people expect that of them.

If you need help breaking old habits, I highly recommend the Boundaries books. Written from a Christian viewpoint, the authors offer empowering insights. If someone can't respect your boundaries, if they only like your *yes* but not your *no,* then that's a sign of an unhealthy relationship.

Break Your Life into Seasons.

Life is a series of seasons, and when you have little control in one season (you are busy until your loved one heals, your home renovation ends, or an issue gets resolved) you can plan for extra rest in the next season.

I have an author friend who rests after every book launch. Once her media interviews and tours are done, she gets off social media and stops writing for six weeks. She journals, reads, takes long walks, and spends extra time with her family. Since writing and launching a book require so much output, she uses this time to refuel.

Another author friend gave me great advice after my first book release. After scheduling back-to-back speaking events, I felt overwhelmed. I didn't realize how drained I'd feel, especially with travel.

I had a deadline for my next book, so I asked my friend how she juggled writing and speaking. She replied, "I do it in seasons. If I'm in a writing season, I don't speak, and if I'm in a speaking season, I don't write."

This made perfect sense, yet I had never considered this strategy. I adopted it in my life, and it has been a game-changer.

Find balance by working in seasons. Lighten your load when you know you will be busy. Some of my happiest seasons came right after my babies were born. For six weeks I felt zero guilt for clearing my calendar, saying *no*, and staying home to focus on them.

As moms we need more guilt-free seasons to pull back or narrow our focus. When life requires more in one area (it's tax season, and you're slammed at work, or a concern with your child has you travelling across the country to get answers) you can simplify in other areas to gain breathing room and head space.

Ecclesiastes 3 says there is a time and a season for every activity under the sun: a time to dance and a time to mourn, a time to embrace and a time to refrain, a time to speak and a time to keep silent. Only God knows what your soul needs, so pray for help in discerning how your seasons should look.

Quit Multitasking.

When my kids were small, multitasking was essential to keeping them alive and cared for at once. I used to tell them "Mommy's not an octopus!" when they pulled on me like a rotisserie chicken, yet an octopus is what I felt like as my arms whirled in constant motion.

Years of multitasking trained my brain to jump around. Now that my girls are older, and I do even *more* mental gymnastics, it affects my concentration. It leaves me mentally exhausted and makes it hard to turn off my brain as thoughts continually churn.

> This daughter needs a prom dress... This one needs more driving time... I have a deadline to meet and feel so stressed... Should I speak at that event? It requires a flight... My child is struggling in math and needs a tutor... She spends a lot of time in her room these days; how can I reach her?... I forgot to set up that ortho appointment... My husband and I need a date night... I sure do miss my friends.

I once prided myself on being a great multitasker, but what I now realize is how multitasking impairs the brain. Surprisingly, we're more productive when we focus. Some research shows that multitasking can reduce productivity as much as 40 percent. It slows you down, causes mistakes, lowers your creativity, and makes you less efficient.

Amy Morin, author of *13 Things Mentally Strong People Don't Do*, says our brains are not nearly as good at handling multiple tasks as we think they are. Multitaskers struggle to tune out distractions more than people who focus on one task at a time.

Rather than jump from one distraction to another, Morin suggests to 1) juggle no more than two tasks at a time and 2) devote your attention fully to one task for twenty minutes before switching to the other.[2]

As a practical example, my friend used to listen to sermons as she did laundry. She carried her laptop on top of her laundry basket as she roamed from room to room. After realizing how she missed key points, she changed her routine. She now sits and watches a sermon without doing anything else. She has relearned how to focus.

Sometimes the best way to find peace and clarity is to do one thing at a time.

Use Your Energy Wisely.

A mom diagnosed with multiple sclerosis said that her doctor's biggest piece of advice was to conserve her energy.

Physically, she couldn't maintain her old schedule. She had to prioritize and be intentional with her time and energy.

This advice applies to all of us. How often do we push ourselves to the max instead of choosing what deserves attention? Just because you *can* do something doesn't mean you *should* do something. Rather than wait for a health crisis, make wise choices now.

Make Sleep a Priority.

God gives us built-in tools to help us relax, which is why breathing strategies work. Sleep is also a tool that keeps us in peak condition.

Making sleep a priority, even if it means accomplishing less in a day, is a cornerstone of self-care.

Thankfully, our society now recognizes sleep as a pathway to wellness. Your body heals during sleep, and according to Medical

News Today, a good night's rest leads to better productivity, performance, and concentration; more energy; more social and emotional intelligence; lower risk for depression, weight gain, and heart disease; better mental functioning; and a stronger immune system.[3]

Even in the corporate world, sleep is a key conversation. Arianna Huffington—after a painful wake-up call in 2007 where she fainted from sleep deprivation and exhaustion, hit her head on her desk, and broke her cheekbone—now uses her transformation to help others change their mind about sleep so they can then change their habits.[4]

Rest in Pockets of Time.

When you are in the thick of parenting, long periods of rest aren't feasible. You can, however, rest in pockets of time.

I used to believe that I had to be productive every minute that my kids were at school. I squeezed in as much work as possible. As they grew up, I incorporated rest into my off-hours to prepare for the chaos after school.

As one mom put it, no matter how relaxed you feel from 8:00 a.m. to 3:00 p.m. with older kids at school, 3:00 p.m. to 8:00 p.m. can undo that peace because once these older kids get home, you work nonstop until bedtime.

This is why I give myself time to sit. I don't rush through a phone call with my dad or a friend. Sometimes I rest during the hour before pickup. Enjoying that calm helps me prepare for the demands soon to come.

My neighbor has four kids, like me. I laughed when she recently told me how she often sits in her car after driving a carpool to catch her breath, return texts, and decompress, because once she walks through the front door, she is "on" again with her boys. My family teases me because I do this too. My car is my second home, and sometimes I sit in the driveway with no agenda at all.

Have People in Your Life Who "Get" You.

A man giving a marriage seminar shared a story about knowing his wife and how that awareness built a happy relationship.

It was their anniversary, so he planned a getaway at a nearby resort. When they arrived at the hotel room, he gave his wife a kiss and a stack of her favorite magazines. He then said he was leaving, because he knew that what his tired spouse really wanted (yet would never verbalize) was a weekend alone in a hotel room, away from noise and her husband's expectations on an anniversary weekend.

Even if you don't have a spouse like this, you can be a friend like this. Create a community where moms notice who is at their wit's end and circle the wagons to help. One day, when you need support or a surprise that speaks to you, you'll be glad you inspired a culture of thoughtful, authentic friendships.

Learn the Art of a Loving "No."

It feels good to say *yes*, but too many *yeses* can get you in trouble. Not every invitation is yours to take, so pray before you commit.

A friend once asked me to speak at her event, and while I believed in her event, my instincts led me to say *no*. When she pressured me to reconsider, I didn't cave because something felt off.

Soon after, another friend of mine lost her husband in a tragedy. It was terrible, and two days before the funeral, I saw a yard sign for my other friend's event. It was scheduled for the same time as the funeral—and I realized then why God prompted that *no*. If I had agreed, I would have had to cancel on her at the last minute.

Only God knows the future, so consult Him as you decide what belongs on your calendar.

Ask Questions.

One way to judge the health of your pace is by asking questions. Consider these:

- *What does my busy life cost me?* If you're so busy that you often feel anxious, impatient, irritated, lonely, defeated, resentful, disconnected, or empty, then it's time to make tweaks or changes. This is also true if you're too busy for basic self-care: if you're always cancelling doctor's appointments, eating junk food on the run, and neglecting your health. Ultimately, this pace leads to burnout.
- *Is it worth it?* When I write a book, I feel extra-stressed for six to eight months. Life is much harder, but it's worth it because 1) God calls me to this work, 2) a short season of pain can create a book with a shelf life of ten years or more, and 3) I've seen firsthand how books help people heal, grow, and find God. Would I take on this extra stress every year? No, because that's not worth it to me, and that's why I spread my books out. Everyone is different, and it's important to know what works for you.
- *Who suffers when I don't pace myself?* My husband gets the short end of the stick with me. He understands when I feel so zapped that I have no energy left for him, but I don't want this, so I've tried to get better about carving out intentional time with him.
- *Do I want to be well?* Obviously, you do, but take it further. What holds you back? What keeps you from eating well, working out, refueling, investing in yourself, and meeting

your core needs? What can you shift around to prioritize these needs?

Give Yourself Room to Grieve—and Permission to Change.

After my father-in-law died, my husband and I felt unmotivated for weeks. Compared to losing a loved one, nothing felt important.

Grief is a process, and while the world will tell you to push through and move on, it is healthier to grieve and heal at an honest pace: to listen to your body, show self-compassion, draw tight with your favorite people, and spend more time in prayer during a season of restoration.

Many women are a Type 2 on the Enneagram personality test (The Helper). A 2 is a caregiver, adept at reading and meeting the needs of others. A 2 is known for their giving spirit.

Grief, however, can temporarily alter key traits like this. An Enneagram 2 friend of mine told me that she hasn't felt like herself since her mother died. She struggles to be the Giver because she's sad and possibly depressed. Her relationship with her husband and her best friend has changed, and while they are both amazing, they can't help her. They're so used to *her* taking care of *them* that the role reversal feels strange.

If you suddenly can't be what you are known for, it's okay. Don't force it and keep pouring out from an empty well. Instead, feed your soul. Fill up on quality inputs, like Scripture, good books, worship music, uplifting movies, encouraging podcasts, a Bible study, and meaningful conversations. Admit your needs and limitations, and let your loved ones support you.

Engage with Nature.

Spending time outdoors is healing, and even sitting on my porch and hearing sounds of nature brings my heart rate down.

Find a "happy place" in nature where God restores your soul. Whether it is walking a favorite trail, sitting on a favorite bench, or spending time at the mountains or the beach, there are places that feel like a deep exhale and awaken a quiet joy inside you.

Decide What Works for You.

I know moms who get off social media when it stirs up discontent with their life. They protect their inner peace, and you can do the same.

I used to respond immediately to every text and email, and it exhausted me. Especially when I was writing, it broke my train of thought. Now I group tasks together. When I have fifteen minutes, I'll respond to all my text messages or emails at once, or I'll catch up on laundry, or I'll make phone calls. Grouping similar tasks together makes demands feel less overwhelming.

Do what works for you. I know moms who do all their laundry on Wednesdays, families that take a Christmas vacation instead of buying gifts, and parents who limit their kids' activities to two at a time. Create a system to facilitate more rest.

Plan Ahead.

What gets planned is what gets done. Since the most important things in life are rarely urgent, it helps to schedule them. Otherwise, demands bleed in.

My husband planned to spend a Saturday with our teenagers. He didn't have a plan, and as their friends invited them over, there was nothing to keep them at home. He let them go, and we learned a lesson about having a plan in place.

Carve out time for rest. Remember how Jesus often went off alone to pray, hear God, and receive comfort and direction. Like you, He couldn't leave His work for long, so He created healthy rhythms. He spent time in solitude with God to prepare for busy seasons, recharge, process grief, gain wisdom, get guidance before big decisions, pour out His heart, and care for His soul. Even before His death, He went off alone to pray and seek comfort from God.

Pray, Wait, and Trust.

God works while you rest, and His timing is perfect. Even if you feel like you'll fall behind, He'll give you the grace to do what must be done.

> Return to your rest, my soul, for the LORD has been good to you.
>
> PSALM 116:7 (NIV)

GIVE YOURSELF GRACE

One thing we realize with age is how we can't beat Father Time.

Our bodies dictate what we can do, and as my daughter learned in AP Biology, our bodies move from a state of *order* to *disorder* as they grow older.

In time, we see the effects or signs of aging. Vital organs lose some function. Hormones change. Muscle and bone loss occurs. Tissues atrophy. Cells lose their ability to function or may function abnormally, mutating and leading to cancer.

You can fight back with health, exercise, and nutrition, but even your best efforts won't give you the vitality of a healthy twenty-year-old. Habits you may have once pulled off, like pulling all-nighters, living on fast food, and bouncing back after a big weekend, will take a bigger toll.

Rather than keep up an old pace that you've outgrown, give yourself grace. Listen to your body, heart, mind, and soul.

The secret to health isn't willpower or trying harder, but rather, being smarter as you navigate the challenges of age.

Aging has mental and psychological perks, thankfully, and making wise choices today sets you up to enjoy them. As a Harvard Medical School professor put it:

> Aging is a continuous process. You can see how people can start to differ in their health trajectory in their 30s, so that by taking good care of yourself early in life you can set yourself on a better course for aging. The best advice I can give is "Take care of your body as though you were going to need it for 100 years," because you might.[5]

Life requires sacrifice, but don't sacrifice your rest. Don't push your body beyond its limits or think that you aren't worthy of downtime. Today's habits set the stage for your future, so find rhythms that keep you well. Remember your long-term goals. And when you feel irritated because your family is having fun without you, consider joining them. A short break may be what you need to exhale, decompress, and reset.

> "Come to me, all who labor and are heavy laden, and I will give you rest."
>
> MATTHEW 11:28 (ESV)

What Rest Models for Your Child

For most of my life, I prided myself on productivity and performance—and had zero value for rest.

It took an "aha" moment with my amazing mom to realize why rest is a foreign concept to me.

Our family of six had just bought a new house and, with my mother's help, we spent five days packing up and cleaning out our existing home. We were exhausted, yet we kept working tirelessly (from daybreak to 10:00 p.m.) to move into our new home.

My mom, a go-getter like me, didn't want to wake my children after bedtime, so she worked in the dark. She thought she was stepping down into a bedroom, only it was a long staircase, and she tumbled down eighteen steps and ended up at the bottom on her back and facing upward, in shock and disoriented.

Upon hearing this sudden, loud, and continuous thunderclap followed by an earth-shattering scream, my husband and I rushed to my mom's side. After an hour of assessing her, we concluded that her lacerations didn't need to be sutured, and she didn't appear to have broken bones.

The next morning, Mom's physician confirmed that, miraculously, she had only broken her pinkie toe. Her black-and-blue body and many lacerations would heal on their own. My mom was bruised, exhausted, and in extreme discomfort, yet when we returned home, she wanted to continue unpacking and getting us settled. She was determined to finish what she started.

That's when it hit me: no wonder it has been so difficult for me to value rest, because I never saw it modeled. Like my mom, I often neglect the rest I need to help the people I love.

Rest doesn't come naturally to me, so I give myself permission. I've learned to find worth in who I am, not what I accomplish. While I value a strong work ethic (and want my children to have one too), I value my health even more. Being mindful of my example keeps me on track. Even if rest feels foreign to me, I hope my kids come to see it as a normal lifestyle rhythm, a habit in our family that they'll want to emulate in their own.

Shannon Runnels Thomas
mom of one son and three daughters

REFLECTION QUESTIONS

1. What is your relationship with busyness? Does it make you feel productive and energized, or drained and overwhelmed?

2. Has your opinion of busyness changed with age? Do you see it as a badge of honor or a sign to scale back?

3. What helps you rest? Do you schedule rest as a life rhythm or postpone it until you hit a stopping point?

4. Have you learned the art of a loving *no*? If not, how can you stop overcommitting?

5. Name three things that are *important* to you and three things that are *urgent*. How can you better prioritize what is important?

6. Have you ever had an "aha" moment regarding rest? Explain.

3

BUILD UPLIFTING FRIENDSHIPS

A Mother Needs to Feel Encouraged

Call it a clan, call it a network, call it a tribe, call it a family. Whatever you call it, whoever you are, you need one. You need one because you are human.

JANE HOWARD, *FAMILIES*[1]

Growing up, I was a great friend. I hosted sleepovers, threw surprise parties, and spent countless hours on the phone talking to my friends.

As a newlywed, I earned the nickname *Julie the Cruise Director* from the TV series *The Love Boat* because I coordinated plans for our couples friends. My husband, Harry, and I had active social lives that kept us busy every weekend.

Things changed as we had children and our family expanded. With each child who came on board, we had less time and energy to pour into friendships. After a long week of work, Harry and I were often so exhausted that we turned down invitations. We became content nesting at home. We stopped doing the play groups and supper clubs that were lifelines when our kids were small.

Slowly, over time, we formed a bubble. We spent our weekends at home: relaxing, catching up, chauffeuring our kids, and hosting their friends. We were happy in our bubble, and since my husband is my best friend, I even went through a phase where I believed that I didn't *need* other friends. My family felt like more than enough to meet my need for community.

Then our kids became teenagers, and we entered a new season of parenting. There was more stress and less family time, and as my oldest daughter turned sixteen and hit the road with her friends, I realized that one day soon, she and her sisters would all leave home. It would be back down to me and Harry. We needed lives beyond our children.

I didn't want to be the clingy parent who lived for their kids to come home. Instead, I wanted to feel excited as they spread their wings and thrilled when they did come home. To be this person in the empty-nester years, I needed good friends and a sense of purpose beyond motherhood. I needed community beyond my home.

Motivated by this, I've spent recent years pouring more time and energy into my friendships. I've quit making excuses, rekindled old friendships, and stayed open to new ones. These efforts have evoked deep feelings of joy and eased the ache of watching my girls grow up. What I didn't realize as I reversed my habits was how much I'd need my friends in a year like 2020.

First, my mom passed away in February. Then, in March, the coronavirus caused a global pandemic. While I felt thankful for the extra time and bonding with my family, this was an unprecedented event, and not even my husband could understand my motherly fears and worries. He couldn't relate to the stress and mental load I carried.

I took many long walks with friends that year, and these conversations were a saving grace that helped me process my challenges, stay connected, and keep a sense of humor.

During this quarantine, I also read a book by former U.S. Surgeon General Dr. Vivek H. Murthy. In his *New York Times* bestseller *Together: The Healing Power of Human Connection in a Sometimes Lonely World,* Dr. Murthy names three "dimensions" of loneliness:

- *Intimate*, or emotional, loneliness is the longing for a close confidante or intimate partner (a deep mutual bond of affection and trust).
- *Relational*, or social, loneliness is the yearning for quality friendships and social companionship and support.

- *Collective* loneliness is the hunger for a network or community of people who share your sense of purpose and interests.

These three dimensions, together, reflect the full range of high-quality social connections that humans need to thrive. Lacking relationships in any dimension can make you lonely, which explains why you may have a supportive marriage yet still feel lonely for friends and community.

Dr. Murthy says healthy relationships are as essential as vaccines and ventilators for our global recovery—and human relationship is as essential as food and water to our well-being.

"Just as hunger and thirst are our body's ways of telling us we need to eat and drink," he writes, "loneliness is the natural signal that reminds us when we need to connect with other people. There's no cause for shame in that. Yet hunger and thirst feel much more acceptable to acknowledge and talk about than loneliness."[2]

Sadly, we live in lonely times. Even before the pandemic, we were living independent and socially disconnected lives. My neighbor and I used to joke that we might go months without seeing each other because her boys and my girls kept us on different paths. Such is the American way: unless your kids overlap on a team or share a common interest, you may go months without seeing your neighbor.

The good news is, we can be intentional. We don't have to leave our friendships to chance, limiting our relationships to whoever crosses our path, and then losing those friendships once the season wraps up or our kids move on to new interests. Real friendships grow deeper roots, and while it takes effort to stay connected, especially if you are on different paths, it is worth it. One day, when our schedules allow more time for friendships, we'll be glad we took the initiative.

After two decades of parenting, I now embrace friendships as a form of self-care. I realize that the older my kids get, the more I need positive peer connections and strong women in my corner. Just as there is a side to my husband that only his buddies bring out, there is a side of me that only my girlfriends can prompt. The world needs this side of me—and it needs this side of you too.

Finding community as females is crucial because we "get" each other. We have similar fears and worries. We crave laughter, humor, and places to vent. We give each other permission to take off our mom hats and relax. We cheer each other on and point out the beautiful (yet hidden) truths that only a woman can see.

Wherever you are now (hungry for friends, happy with friends, or coasting along in a sweet spot where your family feels like enough), consider giving a little extra to your friendships. Having strong ones in place helps sustain you through hard times. They give you a place to fall *and* a place to fall apart. They model good friendships for your children.

It is tempting to neglect your friends when your life is good or when you're exhausted. I have put friends on the back burner for both reasons, only to regret it later. Your need for friendship is real, so don't ignore it. Improve your health by surrounding yourself with uplifting and positive women.

> Two people are better off than one, for they can help each other succeed. If one person falls, the other can reach out and help. But someone who falls alone is in real trouble.
>
> ECCLESIASTES 4:9–10 (NLT)

KNOW WHAT PREVENTS FRIENDSHIPS

I often tell my daughters there is no such thing as a "perfect friend."

In my early teen years, I believed there was, and this mindset made me jump from one BFF to another. What I finally realized is that everyone has strengths and weaknesses, and having a variety of friends took the pressure off any one person having to be my be-all and end-all to everything.

This made me happier, and it made me an easier friend who wasn't impossible to please. Gone were the expectations that nobody could meet.

The goal is not to find perfect companions, but rather, strong companions to journey with: friends who bring out your best, share your goals, and ride your waves with you.

We are all sinful people journeying through a broken world. We all mess up and get it wrong. Nobody ever "masters" relationships, but with trial and error we learn how to be good friends, find good friends, and build healthy friendships.

Here in America we enjoy many blessings, but our culture of achievement can create an inconducive environment for social connection. It can keep us so focused on material goals that we never meaningfully connect.

Following are cultural forces that hinder deep friendships. By being aware, you can avoid these impediments.

Child-Centered Parenting.
We live in an age of child-centered parenting rather than Christ-centered parenting. When our kids become the center of our universe, everything revolves around them, and we, as parents, sacrifice our needs (like adult interaction) to serve them.

Given how all-consuming our kids' schedules can be, it's no surprise that parents stay on a hamster wheel just trying to keep up.

Compare this to our parents' generation, where they kept their social lives and supper clubs because children fit into the existing family order, rather than the family reorganizing around each child. Clearly, family is more important than friends and should be prioritized first, but putting children on an altar has created a false idol with many hidden consequences.

Transactional Relationships.

We also live in an age of "You scratch my back, and I'll scratch yours." Friendships are often based on motives and using people for personal gain.

Parents who desire popularity (for themselves or a child) can socially engineer friendships. Doing this, however, prevents real love, since the opposite of love is using people.[3] As friendships grow transactional, they lose warmth, authenticity, and love.

A Busy Pace.

My husband is Greek and has relatives in Greece. Since 2017, when our family visited the country, we've been enamored with their lifestyle.

In short, they don't live in a rush. They don't own huge, fancy homes that require six-figure salaries and late hours at the office. Their lives are relatively simple, and they treat people like family. On two different tours we did, our guides' mothers made food to share with us. Enjoying a home-cooked meal and dessert made us feel so loved.

The island of Ikaria is a Blue Zone, a region studied by researchers because people live longer, healthier, more disease-free lives (a majority live well past one hundred). Contributing factors are plant-based diets, low stress, a sense of purpose, active lifestyles, a strong sense of family and community, and meaningful connections. Family ties are important, and many homes contain multiple generations where grandparents help raise the grandchildren.[4]

A priest I know worked in Greece for ten years. When I asked him to name the biggest difference compared to America, he noted the pace. In Greece, if you ran into an old friend who you hadn't seen in years, you'd drop everything and have coffee for three hours. In America, you'd exchange numbers and talk about getting together, which might or might not happen. Our calendars stay so full that we rarely have time for impromptu visits.

Lost Villages.

A single mom who works sixty to seventy hours a week told me:

> I grew up with my grandmother at my house every day and on weekends while my dad built his business. My mom could not have raised us without her mother's help. And she didn't work—she was home with us. So for me to work more than full-time and have two kids and be doing it alone, I find myself resenting my mom at times (for not helping) and just wishing and begging for help while beating myself up at how I need to do better. We have lost our community of moms helping other moms without expectation of being paid, or the favor returned, or feeling guilty.

I agree, and I also believe that we need stronger villages for mothers, especially single moms. Many struggle to find community because they are working and feel exhausted, or they feel guilty for leaving their kids at night. Anything that makes them feel supported, seen, and included could mean a lot.

Preconceived Notions.

Many women don't believe in female friendship due to bad experiences. They've bought into ideas about women being mean, catty, and dramatic.

Lumping all women into one category creates a stereotype, and stereotypes are never 100 percent true. While some women are mean and can't be trusted, there are also women who make terrific friends. To write off the entire gender is like throwing out the baby with the bathwater. It creates a self-fulfilling prophecy that hurts us as we search for real friends.

Our world loves to pit females against females, yet when we blindly accept these narratives, we miss opportunities to connect.

Technology.

Technology makes us efficient *and* lazy. Rather than call a friend, we send a text. Rather than catch up over coffee, we scroll through social media. We have gained the ability to function remotely yet lost the art of face-to-face interaction.

Technology also waters down friendship. It makes it appear that we have more real friends than we do. But just because someone takes two seconds to "like" our post does not mean that they'd take off an afternoon to help us in a crisis. Just because we're on a text thread with twenty moms doesn't mean we have one mom we can truly count on. Technology has its benefits, but it can present a false sense of security in friendship.

Disposable Relationships.

In my book *Love Her Well,* I mention the throwaway culture denounced by Pope Francis, a culture where everything is disposable, even relationships, and narcissism makes people incapable of looking beyond themselves. We are quick to connect, disconnect, and block.[5]

Gone are the days of loyal friendships; instead, it is more common to see people dump friends over minor incidents. This creates an atmosphere of every man for himself and stirs up a fear of rejection that brings out the worst in human nature.

Cancel Culture.

Once again, humans are fickle, and never in history has this been more apparent. In this age of cancel culture, where people turn on a dime and crucify anyone who expresses an opposing opinion, we let short-term emotions ruin long-term influence. We lose relationships over petty arguments that won't matter in two years.

Dr. Tim Keller says, "People are messy; therefore, relationships will be messy. Don't be surprised by messiness."[6] Rather than expect perfection, expect your relationships to have some bumps. Expect frustrations, challenges, and glitches. With intentional effort and help from above, we can work through problems. We can help each other grow and thrive.

> "My command is this: Love each other as I have loved you. Greater love has no one than this: to lay down one's life for one's friends."
>
> JOHN 15:12–13 (NIV)

CHOOSE GOOD FRIENDS

In the longest study on happiness ever conducted (eighty years), Harvard researchers discovered that the number-one predictor of lifelong happiness and health is not money or fame, but warm relationships.

"Our relationships and how happy we are in our relationships has a powerful influence on our health," says Robert Waldinger, a professor of psychiatry at Harvard Medical School. "Taking care of your body is important, but tending to your relationships is a form of self-care too. That, I think, is the revelation."

"Loneliness is toxic," Waldinger adds, "and people can feel lonely in relationships and crowds. The people most satisfied in their relationships at age fifty were also the healthiest at age eighty."[7]

Clearly, relationships matter. And if today's relationship choices set the stage for our golden years, why wouldn't we prioritize them? I'll tell you why: because relationships take time, effort, and courage. We're all strapped for time, and we've all been burned by friends who hurt us, yet we can't let the bad apples ruin our hope in humanity. We can't close our hearts to love because of wounds from the past.

God wired us for community, and when we lack community, we feel the void. Rather than dwell in loneliness, we can take action that moves us in the right direction. Here are eight ways to build friendships that go the distance.

1. Work on yourself.

Water seeks its own level, which means that you attract friends similar to you. Women invest a lot of energy in searching for friends and reflecting on how their friends make them feel, but do you ever consider what kind of friend *you* are and how you make your friends feel?

We all have room to grow, and when you point a finger at someone, you have three fingers pointing back at you. Self-reflection can go a long way in elevating your friendship game.

Ephesians 5:1 says, "Be imitators of God..." (ESV). Your most important work on earth will always boil down to relationships, and the key to good relationships is having a faith that inspires you to emulate Him.

2. Be kind.

My friend got a weepy phone call from a young cousin in college who was facing a hard time, yet nobody supported her.

This young cousin had a tough shell and normally prided herself on not needing friends. My friend, a straight shooter, told her, "You can't go around being mean to people and then expect them to be there for you when you need them."

This sounds like common sense, but for many people, it is not.

We live in a mean world where women and girls are encouraged to be hard-core. On a good day this may work, but when the chips are down, loneliness will surface. Kindness is often perceived as weakness, but it is really a sign of strength. It takes self-control to be kind when others are not.

My biggest prerequisite for choosing friends is kindness, and it has never steered me wrong. I can invite any friends to spend time together and know they will get along. Good people like good people, and the best thing to have in common is a caring heart.

3. Initiate.

One mistake that we make in friendships is expecting others to make the first move. But the fact is, *you* have the power to start a conversation, introduce yourself, plan a fun adventure, host a party, and put yourself in social positions.

Don't be scared to do the inviting, take the first step, or start the dynamics that build community. Even if someone says *no*, you'll eventually find someone who says *yes*.

4. Make plans.

Again, what gets planned is what gets done. Since relationships are rarely urgent, you must carve out time for them; otherwise, they'll fall through the cracks.

My sister-in-law takes an annual beach trip with her best friends from college. They've done this trip for thirty years, leaving an open invitation for whoever can make it. I know another girl who does her annual girls' trip on Mother's Day weekend. They are all home by Sunday afternoon to celebrate with their families.

My friend's mother hosts sleepovers at the lake with her friends, and my friend Jennifer once hosted her college friends in her home while her husband took the kids out of town. They stayed in their PJs all weekend, talking, laughing, and enjoying good food and wine.

Even if you can't do a girls' trip, consider a mother-son or a mother-daughter getaway. Combine it with a fun concert or a college visit to enjoy extra time with your child, their friends, and moms who you enjoy.

5. Don't keep score.

Relationships work best when both people are Givers. Rarely, however, is the giving equal because circumstances change.

I once received an email from a woman regarding a friendship struggle. Her good friend had just discovered her husband's infidelity, and she asked for space to work through this pain with God. This woman was missing her friend and feeling neglected because her efforts to reach out weren't reciprocated. She asked for my opinion.

I said that while friendships need a healthy balance of give-and-take, there are some seasons where people don't have much to give. I have friends who have walked through infidelity, and it took all their energy to get out of bed and care for their kids. They had nothing left over for friends.

I advised this woman to rely on *other* friends for her needs. Then, she could turn around and give extra love and support to her hurting friend without any expectations in return.

Sometimes the best gift you can give a friend is to take the pressure off, to not get upset if a text isn't returned or an invitation isn't accepted because they're getting back on their feet and, until they are, you'll extend extra grace and not keep score.

6. Don't struggle alone.

Today's parents were raised by parents who largely followed *The Amy Vanderbilt Complete Book of Etiquette*. Transparency was not the norm, and in many homes, awkward issues weren't discussed. Problems and dysfunctions got swept under the rug as everyone pretended that they didn't exist.

But keeping secrets makes you lonely, and if you don't turn to people for help, you're likely to turn to other comforts, like alcohol, food, or drugs.

After my mom passed away, I didn't know how to mourn her. I tried to remember how she handled the loss of her mother, and I couldn't, so I decided to let my daughters see me grieve so they'd have a blueprint in their lives.

When one daughter overheard me talking to a friend, she said, "Wow, Mom, you're so honest!" I'd just told my friend that I was doing okay after a breakdown earlier, and I explained to my daughter how letting my friends in allowed them to help me. She nodded and understood.

We all have struggles, and with depression and anxiety levels at all-time highs, there is too much at stake to fight your struggles alone. Let your friends help you, and they'll come to you when they need help too.

7. Know who is good for you.

I once went on a girls' trip that drained me. The entire weekend consisted of griping and gossip, and while I've been guilty of both, I felt the toxicity the whole way home. I promised to not put myself in that position again.

Real friends inspire the best version of you. They may call your bluff, but they'll speak the truth in love. They're a source of comfort, not stress. They cushion the pain of the world.

You will never reach full potential surrounded by the wrong people, so choose wisely where you invest time. Choose friends who build you up and speak life.

8. Plug in.

Shared passions bring automatic friendships. As a fellow author once told me, when a writer meets another writer, you go from zero to eight on the get-to-know-you scale. You skip over pleasantries and connect on a deeper level.

Whatever your passion is (rescuing dogs, water sports, cooking, fitness, marathons, book clubs, gardening, medicine, sewing), plug into that community. Remember how people are hungry to connect and find others who share their interests.

Most people can count their best friends on one hand, and if you have that, you're lucky. **A Sugarland song talks about how there are some hands you *shake* and some hands you *hold*.** Casual friends are the hands you shake. They last for a season, maybe a few seasons. Committed friends are the hands you hold. They last for a lifetime and become your sisters of the heart.

One of life's greatest joys is to have amazing friends and transporting conversations that make you lose track of time. In these moments, life feels good and makes sense. Even if past friendships let you down, search for friendships like this. Open your heart to possibilities, and anchor your confidence in the God who inspires genuine love.

> So encourage each other and build each other up, just as you are already doing.
>
> 1 Thessalonians 5:11 (nlt)

REACH OUT AND RECONNECT

My best lessons in friendship came during my loneliest season of friendship.

As a newlywed in a new city, I started at square one. I got invited to many parties, yet I didn't have any deep connections. Every girl I knew already had a best friend, and since many grew up together, I felt like an outsider as they shared childhood stories.

After one girls' night out, I came home and cried to my husband. I told him how I just couldn't compete with friends who had known each other since they were in diapers and taken baths together at two years old. *Everyone was kind, but nobody needed me like I needed them.* It took me six months of effort and accepting every invitation that came my way to finally get my bearings.

My turning point came when I met Mary Alice, who had just moved back to town. We immediately clicked and became close friends. From that friendship we grew other friendships and expanded our circle. When my husband and I moved four years later, we were genuinely sad to leave these friends who had become our family.

Looking back, I realize that my problem was insecurity. I had a void in my heart that longed to be filled with the gift of female connection. Rather than let it happen naturally, I tried to force it. I was so eager to find my place that I was petrified of making mistakes.

What should have been fun—meeting new people—had me walking on eggshells because I couldn't let down my guard, relax, and be myself.

Today, I'm thankful for that dry season of friendship. Among other things, I learned

- what it feels like to be an outsider—and what a simple invitation (like going on a walk) can mean to a woman who hasn't found her people yet,
- how to be proactive and not wait for friendships to magically happen,
- how loneliness can crop up even if you're happy in your marriage,
- how nobody thrives in every season, and that's okay because dry seasons teach you to be kind and inclusive (and to reflect on what kind of friend you've been),
- how to tell the difference between acquaintances and lifelong friends,
- why it's worth bending over backward for lifelong friends, because they're hard to find, and
- why one true friend is worth her weight in gold.

Real friends offer a healthy escape and recharge our batteries. They make us feel young again and remind us of who we are. They don't judge us or our kids when we have a bad day, and they don't have expectations like family. They aren't stuck with us like family, so when they stay despite our shortcomings, it's affirming.

Being loved by a friend helps us love ourselves.

Don't wait until your children are older, or until you have

more free time, to nurture your friendships. You need good friends now as you learn to "be the adult." You and I are in a season where we must be the strong and reliable ones, and we can't do this alone. We need the strength and moral support of women who rally for us.

Think about the friends you've known over time who brought out your best. Who inspires you? Who would be on your doorstep in a crisis? Who loved you so deeply in the past that the bond is still there?

Whoever these friends are, reach out and reconnect. Invest in these relationships. You don't want to look back in twenty years and realize that you gave your best efforts to short-term friends and acquaintances. You don't want to settle for pleasant relationships when rich relationships are in reach.

Embrace your old friends, and leave room for new friends too. Sometimes the best friendships of all are the ones you've yet to make.

As iron sharpens iron, so a friend sharpens a friend.
PROVERBS 27:17 (NLT)

What Uplifting Friendships Model for Your Child

The summer before seventh grade, I lost my mom to cancer. Although I had friends, it wasn't anyone my age who sustained me: it was my grandmother, my aunt, and my mom's wonderful friends.

They were my lifeline.

My mom was an amazing woman of God and a dear friend to many. She had Christian friendships, the kind that can only come from God, and these women sat at her bedside as she battled cancer. After my mom passed away, these women invested in me, shaped me, and loved me.

In high school, as I formed my own friendships, I was blessed by these women and by the mothers of my friends. (One was particularly influential. She was like a second mom to me, and I adore her to this day.) These moms made sure that I had what I needed—nails done for prom, bedding for my college dorm, recommendation letters for sorority rush—and were always available. Also in high school, my dad remarried a precious woman. At the time I couldn't recognize what a gift she'd be to me, so I pushed her away and relied more on my friends' mothers.

What these incredible women taught me is that to have good friends, you must be a good friend. Because my mom understood this, I reaped the benefits. Good friends show up and commit for the long haul, even when it's not convenient. I was shocked when my friend's mom drove a long way to attend my father's funeral. When I told her, "I can't believe you came!" she replied, "This is what you do for the people that you love." Her remark has always stuck with me and been my mantra ever since.

I place great value on teaching my children how to be a good friend. I've experienced that lifeline firsthand, and after having my mom's friends plus my high school friends' mothers love on me through difficult years—taking me under their wing and treating me like their own—I try to pay it forward. These women modeled friendship perfectly. What a gift to know women like this and see the ripple effects still today.

Andrea Paterson Goodson
mom of three sons and one daughter

REFLECTION QUESTIONS

1. Do you think friendships are a form of self-care? Why or why not?

2. How have your friendships changed (for better or for worse) since college and since your early days of motherhood? Do you put in more effort or less effort now?

3. What did your loneliest season of friendship teach you? Would you do anything differently?

4. Women often give up on friendships after painful experiences. What pain is holding you back or making you hide your vulnerable side?

5. Name your three best friends ever. Are they still in your life? If not, should you reach out?

6. Has friendship ever created a lifeline for you? Explain.

4

CONQUER STRESS AND ANXIETY WITH TRUTH

A Mother Needs to Feel Empowered

Other than showing your child love and affection, managing your own stress is the best thing you can do to be an effective parent.

SISSY GOFF, *RAISING WORRY-FREE GIRLS*[1]

My friend's sixteen-year-old daughter called her from school, panicked and stressed.

"Mom, you've got to check me out! Everybody is saying how hard this history test is. I know I'll fail it. Please come get me so I don't have to take it today!"

Immediately my friend knew that her daughter had spent time in the Mall. The Mall is our high school's common area where the students congregate. Oftentimes, they make each other panic as they discuss the difficulty of their classes or share their grades. My friend often warned her daughter to beware of the "Mall Mentality," and this was exactly why.

"I'm not going to check you out," her mom calmly replied, "because you're ready for this test. Get out of the Mall and go to the library to clear your head. You have studied, and you know the material. I promise you'll do fine."

Her daughter wasn't convinced, but she listened to her mom. She made an A on that history test, and two years later, this straight-A student was named a National Merit Finalist. She won a full scholarship to the college of her choice. She graduated with top honors.

Clearly, she is an intelligent student who had prepared for this test, so why did she suddenly doubt herself? And what does it say for the rest of us when even the brightest people, the ones whom you would never imagine getting rattled, lose sight of their ability to handle challenges?

In some way, we can all relate. We all have "Malls" in our life that trigger self-doubt and panic. Even when we work hard, even when we leave home feeling confident, it only takes a voice or two to stir up worry, stress, or anxiety.

As we listen to the wrong voices, from the critic in our head to the doomsayers around us, we forget the truths we know deep down. We let our minds spiral into hopeless places. We tune into the voices of people (or the enemy) rather than the quiet whispers of God.

Thankfully, God knows our struggles. He understands how we second-guess ourselves and let our confidence swing. Too often, we let the influence of the Mall Mentality make us emotional, not rational. We accept a group mindset without considering what we believe.

Some stress in life is healthy, helping us rise to the occasion, build resilience, and overcome a challenge or dangerous situation, but more common is the unhealthy stress that, left unchecked, can develop into anxiety. Both stress and anxiety have similar symptoms and are part of the body's fight-or-flight reaction. The difference is that stress tends to be short term and in response to a recognized threat. Anxiety can linger and may not have a clear trigger. While stress is the body's reaction to a threat, anxiety is the body's reaction to stress.[2]

Even if you've never wrestled with anxiety, you probably know someone who has. Anxiety disorders are the most common mental illness in the United States today, affecting 40 million adults age eighteen or older (18 percent of the population).[3] Most of us have felt anxious feelings. We know what it's like to feel stable and confident one minute—and panicked the next.

When this happens, remember these truths:

1. Both stress and anxiety throw you into fight-or-flight mode. They activate your amygdala, the fear center of your brain, which is primitive and emotional.

2. A fight-or-flight reaction is necessary for real danger (like when a bear is chasing you), but with stress and anxiety, it can make you overreact and overestimate the problem.

3. Proper breathing can calm you. The 4–7–8 breathing technique, touted by Dr. Andrew Weil, calms your nervous system (helping it break out of the fight-or-flight response triggered by fear) and relaxes your body. Simply inhale through your nose for four seconds, hold your breath for seven seconds, and exhale through your mouth for eight seconds.[4]

4. What also calms you is letting your prefrontal cortex, the control center of your brain, stay in charge so your amygdala doesn't take over. Your prefrontal cortex assesses the threat and logically determines an appropriate response. It tells the amygdala whether the alarm is justified.

5. Anxiety escalates when there is an "amygdala hijack," when you feel threatened and afraid, and your amygdala activates the fight-or-flight response. Normally, your frontal lobes take control (and bring reason into the situation), but in this case, the amygdala disables them and hijacks control. Without your frontal lobes, you can't think clearly, make rational decisions, or control your responses.[5]

A physiological reaction to anxiety is scary, and the only way to fight it is to face it. While some people find strategies on their own, others enlist the help of a counselor. Counselors teach you how to "sit with anxiety," feel the discomfort, and talk yourself through it (like my friend did for her daughter). They give words to complicated feelings. They help you find outlets to redirect your anxiety, such as art, writing, music, journaling, meditation, prayer, and time in nature. They determine whether medical assistance may be needed.

Most importantly, counselors foster self-awareness. Being self-aware helps you know your triggers and work toward a rational place. This place matters because once your mind settles, you become capable of hearing truth. Your basic need for safety is taken care of, and now that you can think clearly, you can remember God's promises and discern His whispers to you.

> "My sheep listen to my voice; I know them, and they follow me."
>
> JOHN 10:27 (NIV)

TRUST TRUTH OVER EMOTION

One of the loudest "Malls" in my life is social media.

I have mixed feelings about social media because, on one hand, I love it. I like keeping up with friends, making new friends, and sharing my writing across the globe. Thanks to social media, I've been invited to publish books and speak to audiences. I've seen the upside of this platform, and I'm aware of the doors it can open.

On the other hand, social media messes with my psyche. Some days I feel like I am doing everything wrong as a mom and a writer. I compare myself to moms who are better homemakers or simply more fun. I read the work of more talented writers and suddenly hate my writing style.

In these moments, I go from self-confidence to self-criticism. Rather than embrace the unique person I'm meant to be, I feel an urge to reinvent myself and be more like the people I most admire.

Social media also confuses me with information overload. As an eager student of life, I absorb it all (stories, photos, opinions, news) because I like to learn and stay informed. I enjoy keeping a pulse on our culture and engaging in relevant conversations.

On one level this is good, but too often I take in too much. I get overly stimulated and mentally exhausted. My head starts to spin and short-circuit. I struggle to hear God over the chatter of voices. I forget the truths I know deep down.

Last year, I had an epiphany while skimming a popular Facebook page for parents of teenagers. When one mom asked for advice on helping her college-age daughter handle a bad roommate, more than 700 moms replied. They all had strong opinions and conflicting advice.

As I scanned the comments, I wondered, *Who is this woman supposed to listen to? Everyone thinks they have the perfect answer, so who is right?* It hit me then why we need God, one central source of truth. Without Him, we confuse each other. We become the blind leading the blind, instructing each other based on feelings and experiences.

Ten years ago, we may have gotten three conflicting opinions, but today we can get 700. No wonder we're more confused than previous generations! Living in the digital age gives us access to every opinion that ever existed. It makes it extra tricky to separate *truth* from *emotion*.

The enemy desires this. He wants our minds foggy since God desires the opposite. God is a God of peace, not confusion (1 Corinthians 14:33). He brings order, not disorder. We crave knowledge, and we have a world of knowledge at our fingertips, yet what we really need is wisdom. Wisdom comes from God;

it comes from trusting the truths planted inside our heart and imparted through the Holy Spirit.

Sometimes I find wisdom on social media. On Facebook, for instance, I recently saw this: "Ships don't sink because of the water *around* them. Ships sink because of the water that gets *in* them. Don't let what's happening around you get inside you and weigh you down."

It was inspired by Isaiah 43:2 (NLT): "When you go through deep waters, I will be with you. When you go through rivers of difficulty, you will not drown. When you walk through the fire of oppression, you will not be burned up; the flames will not consume you."

God is present, even in a crisis, and the way to stay afloat is to not let external factors (like human voices or opinions) seep in and shake your confidence in Him.

This is easier said than done, but thankfully, the Bible is packed with truths to help us. God is sovereign, and promises like these help us tune out distractions:

- God is the Alpha and the Omega, the First and the Last, the Beginning and the End. (Revelation 22:13)
- God's perfect love drives out fear. (1 John 4:18)
- Even when you enter impossible new territory and can't see a way forward, God will do a new thing, making a way in the wilderness and streams in the desert. (Isaiah 43:18–19)
- God gives strength to the weary and power to the weak. (Isaiah 40:29)
- The hope of Jesus is an anchor for your soul. (Hebrews 6:19)
- You can find joy in trials because the testing of your faith produces perseverance and spiritual maturity. (James 1:2–4)

- No weapon formed against God's children will prosper. (Isaiah 54:17)
- You can rejoice in suffering because suffering produces perseverance; perseverance, character; and character, hope. (Romans 5:3–4)
- If you remain faithful to Jesus' teachings, then you will know the truth, and the truth will set you free. (John 8:31–32)
- God hears your prayers and answers them wisely. You can bring your prayers to Him with confidence, knowing that those who ask will receive, those who seek will find, those who keep knocking will get doors opened. (Matthew 7:7)
- God will not always remove thorns from your life. He may allow a struggle (like anxiety) to keep you humble. Even so, you can boast of your weaknesses so that Christ's power rests on you. When you are weak, He is strong. (2 Corinthians 12:7–10)

Truth is not about majority opinion, what's trending in the news, or what gains traction on Facebook. It isn't decided by humans or the "Malls" of your life.

The truth we have today is the same truth that existed when Jesus walked the earth. It is reliable, unchanging, and comforting. It is not a "thing," but rather, a person: Jesus. In a world that has lost its way, where we often feel stressed or anxious because we don't know who to trust or what to believe, we have wisdom that has stood the test of time, truth that elevates what is real.

> Jesus told him, "I am the way, the truth, and the life. No one can come to the Father except through me."
>
> JOHN 14:6 (NLT)

"PRAY, HOPE, AND DON'T WORRY"

You probably have many sources of stress and anxiety as a mother.

One, family life is hard. From managing schedules to stress levels, you juggle more balls and demands than the moms who walked before you.

Two, there is never enough of you to go around. There is *one* of you caring for *multiple* people. Even on your best days, you are shorthanded.

Three, you care. It would be easier to not care, but as it stands, you worry about the big and little heartaches, challenges, and battles that your children face. You know their life details, which leads to more concerns.

Four, our culture expects perfection—and nothing less.

Five, you get bombarded with images of every mom on the planet. Comparisons or guilt about what you "should do" or "could do" can make your mothering feel inadequate.

Six, you are intuitive. You pick up on changes in moods and behavior that suggest your loved one has an issue. This is a gift, yet it also adds to your plate.

Seven, you constantly make decisions based on limited information, and you worry that a bad decision will ruin your child's future.

And eight, your worry lingers. You can't compartmentalize it or turn it off. My friend and I just laughed about the difference between her and her husband. After she expressed a concern about their son, they had a serious conversation. They agreed this needed attention. Two minutes later, she heard her husband whistling around their house. He had moved on, yet she was still worried. Maybe you can relate, as I certainly do!

A counselor once told me that if we don't put our anxiety into something higher than ourselves, then we'll try to

micromanage it. Here, I believe, is where we get sidetracked. Anxiety comes when we envision a future without Jesus.[6] It comes when we wrongly assume it all depends on us, so we panic and try to control things so our nightmares don't come true.

In the process, we focus on our limitations rather than God's power. We make it about us, not Him. We narrow our gaze to an unhealthy extreme.

Anxiety and stress are real, and, as moms, we must learn to handle them for our health *and* the sake of our children. In a famous study based on decades of research, Dr. Robert Epstein named the most important qualities of good parenting, the skills most vital to bringing up healthy, happy, and successful kids.

Predictably, giving love and affection was number one on the list. *The big surprise was number two on the list: handling stress as a parent.* Both number two and number three (relationship skills, having a good relationship with your spouse/significant other/coparent and other people) are more helpful to your parenting than some child-focused behaviors.

Dr. Epstein defined stress management as taking steps to reduce stress for yourself and your child, practicing relaxation techniques, and promoting positive interpretations of events.[7]

Like my friend in the opening story, we help our children by reframing a situation with truth and logic. *If my friend didn't have the skills to manage her own moments of panic, she might have panicked with her daughter and prompted a different (and less favorable) outcome.*

As mothers, our stress and anxiety spill over to our family. I say this not to guilt-trip anyone but to remind us why mental health deserves attention. Personally, I'm easily rattled. Anxiety creeps up on me, and I doubt I'll be cured on this side of heaven.

While I wish I didn't feel anxious, I also see this as a desirable difficulty. Anxiety has forced me to grow a deeper faith. It propels me toward God, because after years of searching for peace, nothing soothes my heart like trusting and resting in Him.

When you feel stressed or anxious, trust the bigger truths. Remember how God has equipped you and chosen you to be your child's mom. Regardless of what your inner critic or the "Malls" around you say, you can do hard things. You can rise to the challenge before you. You can

- stay strong for your family,
- survive a season of hell,
- recover from a failure or rejection,
- face heartache and pain,
- sit with unpleasant thoughts and emotions,
- have dreaded conversations,
- make amends,
- help your child face adversity,
- handle hate or criticism,
- love yourself,
- see some trials as desirable difficulties,
- turn over a new leaf,
- make guilt-free decisions,
- do your part today, and trust God to take care of tomorrow.

Saint Padre Pio said, "Pray, hope, and don't worry."[8] These simple words replace doubt and fear with trust and obedience. They remind us to give the burden of worry, stress, and anxiety to our loving Father, who accepts it all.

> Don't worry about anything; instead, pray about everything.
> Tell God what you need, and thank him for all he has done.
>
> PHILIPPIANS 4:6 (NLT)

What Conquering Stress and Anxiety with Truth Models for Your Child

Like most women, I worry, but my anxiety spiked to new levels when my husband David faced a crisis in 2019.

What started as a normal night in our small town, watching our son's basketball game, led to a sudden headache for David that got so severe we went to the ER. Our doctor friend studied the scan, and then calmly broke the news that David had a brain bleed and would need a helicopter airlift to the nearest medical center.

As I hugged my emotional husband, he whispered, "I love you, and I am so sorry." Given the uncertainty, David knew the burden this placed on me and our teenage sons.

Walking out of that hospital, my knees buckled, and I fell into the arms of two of my best friends. They literally held me up as reality hit. What would I tell our boys? What if their dad didn't make it through the night and get to say good-bye? Who would care for them while I stayed at the hospital? How would I raise three sons if David died or was disabled?

The next two weeks were a whirlwind of tears, fears, and prayer warriors. David had a 50/50 chance of survival and a 50/50 chance of disability if he made it. Emotionally, it was terrible, but spiritually, it was miraculous. The hands and feet of Jesus came profoundly alive as friends from every season of life carried us. My best friends rotated staying with me, and I had no idea how desperately I'd need them at night. That is when Satan attacked my thoughts with worries and fear.

My sweet friends spoke truth over me and prayed fiercely. They calmed my anxiety when my mouth felt too paralyzed to speak. Looking back, I think of Romans 8:26 (NIV): "In the same way, the Spirit helps us in our weakness. We do not know what we ought to pray for, but the Spirit himself intercedes for us through wordless groans." Even when we can't pray, the Holy Spirit finds ways to pray for us.

God chose to heal David after a long, hard recovery. At first our sons struggled to see their strong and masculine dad suddenly weak and relearning to walk. Since then, however, we've seen God's faithfulness repeatedly— like when our oldest son in college considered going into physical therapy after watching what they did for David. Moments like this are humbling. They remind me how God wastes nothing, and by choosing to trust Him, we open the door to new blessings in our life and the lives of our children.

Jill Barrett Partridge
mother of three sons

REFLECTION QUESTIONS

1. Name a "Mall" in your life that triggers stress or anxiety. What truths can you repeat when it messes with your psyche?

2. Have you ever experienced an "amygdala hijack," flying into fight-or-flight mode instead of logically thinking through a fear or threat? Looking back, what would you do differently?

3. Does social media ever take you from self-confidence to self-criticism? Does listening to the world's opinions make it harder to hear God's voice?

4. What are your three most dominant emotions (for example: fear, anger, anxiety, joy, excitement, impatience, contempt, frustration, sadness, sympathy)? How do they color/rule your life and outlook?

5. Are you surprised that handling your stress as a parent is the *second* most important skill to raising healthy, successful children? Does this motivate you to cultivate this skill for your family's sake?

6. Has a crisis ever spiked your anxiety? If so, what role did truth play in regaining control of your mind?

5

CHOOSE JOY

A Mother Needs to
Feel Comforted

*Joy does not simply happen to us. We have
to choose joy and keep choosing it every day.
It is a choice based on the knowledge that we
belong to God and have found in God our
refuge and our safety and that nothing, not
even death, can take God away from us.*

HENRI NOUWEN[1]

It was the Friday of Mother's Day weekend and my mother was sick. Her health had taken a sudden nosedive, and though doctors had run a series of tests, no one could pinpoint the cause.

My siblings and I had cried all week. My dad seemed to have aged about twenty years. No one said it out loud, but we sensed this might be the end. She was on the brink of death.

While my kids were at school Friday, I stayed at the hospital. My mother was unresponsive, and as I saw how it took several nurses to change her clothes and move her limp body, my heart broke. Where was my strong, capable, determined mother? Who was this woman too helpless to take care of herself?

I expected her to bounce back, to dig deep and recover like the Steel Magnolia she was, but her condition looked bleak. Besides feeling sad, I felt cheated. Losing a mother on Mother's Day weekend was a cruel irony. I wasn't sure how I'd ever get over that.

Around lunchtime, my phone alarm sounded, signaling my time to leave. I had been invited to a Mother's Day Tea for my youngest daughter, Camille, who was in kindergarten at the time. Normally, I loved these teas, but this one I dreaded. I didn't feel like faking joy. My eyes were swollen, and my heart was in a vulnerable place.

But as we moms do, I pushed through my feelings and made myself go. I'm so glad I did, not only for Camille's sake, but also for myself.

As you might imagine, the kindergartners were running wild as I entered the classroom. They were thrilled to see their mothers and high on the anticipation of eating cupcakes after their performance.

They laughed, sang, and grinned from ear to ear as they thanked us for taking care of them. The classroom overflowed with energy, youthfulness, and life—and I couldn't help but notice the striking contrast this presented to the hospital scene that I had left.

I had gone from a place of illness to a place of vitality, a place where people were nearing the end of their journey to a place where journeys were just beginning.

Out of the blue, my heart swelled with new emotions. Once again that day, I held back tears, only these were *happy* tears. I needed this hour of joy on an incredibly sad day. I needed to spend time with rambunctious six-year-olds whose joy could not be contained.

In this moment, I felt God's goodness. I understood how He really does know and meet our needs. As I looked at Camille (my fourth child, the surprise baby who I felt ill-equipped to have because I was so overwhelmed as a mom of three), I realized that God knew, even as I cried throughout her pregnancy, how He'd use Camille to restore me on this particularly trying day.

All my doubts about having a fourth child vanished once Camille was born, and as I'd done countless times since that day, I thanked God for this little girl who I did not have the foresight to pray for. Like her sisters, she was an undeserved gift, and at this Mother's Day Tea, I felt overwhelmingly aware of this.

I also felt guilt for feeling joy while my mom was sick. There was a strange tension in my heart unlike any I'd known before. How could I feel intense joy and deep sadness on the same day? How could I reconcile the conflicting emotions without letting one overshadow the other?

I wondered if this was what "adulting" looked like, and if

I'd entered a new stage of life where letting opposite emotions peacefully coexist was the only way to move forward.

Thankfully, my mother survived that difficult weekend. She never walked again or fully rebounded, but she hung on for four more years and showed remarkable resilience. She had more close calls where we wondered if she'd make it, and with each setback I looked for silver linings. When heartache tries to drag us into the abyss of a black hole, silver linings ground us. They keep grief from engulfing us.

Even in trials and times of sorrow, your heart can feel joy. These moments are made possible through God's supernatural grace. Feel your pain, but fight for your joy. Don't let people or events steal your joy or lead you to mistakenly believe that your joy is over.

> May the God of hope fill you with all joy and peace as you trust in him, so that you may overflow with hope by the power of the Holy Spirit.
>
> ROMANS 15:13 (NIV)

MINE YOUR LIFE FOR JOY

A young mom in my neighborhood told me that her favorite parenting advice came from an older mother who said:

> *Whatever season your children are in, enjoy it. Don't wish it away. When you wish away the hard parts of a season, you also wish away the good parts.*

Isn't this true? When your toddler drives you nuts, and you wish the toddler years were over because you're tired of temper tantrums, ear infections, and constant chasing, you're also wishing away sweet snuggles on the couch, exuberant hugs and kisses, the wonder on their face as they talk about Santa Claus or Mickey Mouse, and how irresistibly cute they look in their Superman and Disney princess pajamas.

Moments that make your heart sing only last for a phase, and one day, you'll miss them.

In a similar vein, finding joy is about embracing the good within the hard. It takes effort and awareness. We often miss joy because

1. we're fantasizing about the day when life will be easier,
2. we're so busy keeping up that we get tunnel vision and limited perception,
3. joy is buried and requires digging,
4. we expect joy to come with an elaborate bang, and
5. life has hurt us, hardened us, or blinded us to seeing what is praiseworthy and right.

Joy can feel elusive as you deal with the heartache of a broken world. It can seem like a part of the past that you'll never recapture again. The truth, however, is that your best days are still ahead. Perfect joy doesn't exist on this side of heaven, but it does exist in our final destination—the joy of eternity that God created us to run toward.

As Paul wrote in Philippians 3:13–14 (NLT), "No, dear brothers and sisters, I have not achieved it, but I focus on this one thing: Forgetting the past and looking forward to what lies ahead, I press on to reach the end of the race and receive the heavenly prize for which God, through Christ Jesus, is calling us."

How does this look in real life? How do you view today's

problems through the lens of joy and promise? Here are some ways to find joy and bridge reality with eternity.

Grieve What Was (and Celebrate What Is).

Losses are painful, and giving yourself the space to feel a loss, even years later, is healing. It is also healing to remember that grief is an expression of love. We grieve for the people we love.

My friend Beth felt a huge loss after her mother died. Christmas triggered memories, and decorating her tree was particularly hard because her mom had given her many ornaments with pictures of special events, such as their wedding, their first dog, and their kids at the beach.

To give space to her grief, Beth created a ritual. Every year as her family decorates their Christmas tree, they set aside the ornaments from Beth's mom. Then, after the kids go to bed, Beth pours herself a glass of wine, sits alone in front of the tree, and cries. She hangs her mom's ornaments and releases her feelings. This is Beth's way of saying, "I'm going to remember her and let myself get upset so the sadness doesn't linger, and I can enjoy the holidays with my kids." It helps her grieve what used to be.

Be honest about your feelings. Remember that tears shed over a loved one simply prove how important they were to you. Love has no time limits, and creating rituals to honor the past enables you to celebrate what you have today.

Laugh.

Laughter is healing, especially during heartache. Years ago, my friend lost her home in a fire. As she stood on the street, watching with neighbors as firemen tried to extinguish the flames and save her greatest treasures, she saw them bring out a large oil portrait of her son. She never liked this portrait because it didn't look like her son, and it wasn't the best quality. Her closest friends were aware of this. As the crowd cheered, assuming the firemen had accomplished an amazing feat by saving this portrait, her close friend leaned in and whispered a joke to lament its survival. This moment of comic relief came exactly when my friend needed it most.

Give Thanks.

Most people aren't naturally grateful, and that's why a habit of gratitude matters. Even if your life unravels, you can thank God for His character and good plans for you. You can guard your heart against cynicism by giving thanks for what you have.

We all take for granted the blessing of health. It's been said that a healthy person has a thousand wishes, while an unhealthy person has only one wish. There are always parts of you to praise God for: eyes that see, legs that walk, a mind that thinks, a heart that loves. Even the ability to work and take care of your family is a blessing worth acknowledgment.

Joy comes as you remember what God has done for you and the people you love. Reflect on your blessings (a son who loves you and gives the best hugs, a daughter who lights up the room, a husband or best friend who has your back, parents who show up for you, a boss who believes in you, a special talent, a determined spirit), and know that every good gift comes from above.

Erase the "Perfect" Picture in Your Head.

Our world conditions us early to be perfectionists.

When we are young, perfection seems attainable, yet as we begin careers, get married, have kids, and grow up, we learn ugly truths about ourselves and the world. We get humbled by people and events beyond our control. We despair when life falls short of how it's supposed to be. We resent anyone who interrupts our perfect plan. We fear looking imperfect. We lose peace, connection, and joy.

This is no way to live, and what all of us must decide is whether to keep chasing a perfect life or to embrace the imperfect life we have.

I once heard a great sermon from Father Bob Sullivan about life lessons from baseball. He said that in baseball, a batting average of .300 is considered excellent. Errors are accepted, and even the best athletes strike out. In real life, however, we reject the idea of only hitting three balls out of ten. We expect perfection—and nothing less.

But could that be our problem? If we applied baseball's philosophy to life, would it relieve the pressure we feel, destigmatize failure, reframe disappointments, and help us move forward? I believe so. We are imperfect humans in an imperfect world, but if we learn from each challenge and setback, we can't be defeated.

More important than creating a perfect life is creating a meaningful life. This brings more joy and builds deeper and more rewarding relationships. Make meaning your goal, and joy will come even on your off days.

Create a Life You Don't Long to Escape.

The average American spends 200 hours a year (equal to 24 workdays) daydreaming about vacation.[2]

While I'm as guilty as anyone of dreaming of blissful reprieves, it doesn't speak well for our culture that we spend an inordinate amount of time longing to escape our busy lives.

We live in a work-hard, play-hard society. We're pushed to be workaholics and not get left behind. But when busyness creates a lifestyle that requires a vacation to relax, something is wrong. You choose your pace, so find one that leaves room for joy without having to leave home.

Love the Simple Things.

In her article "Dear Teenagers, Here's How to Protect Your Emotional Well-Being," Dr. Lisa Damour discusses the upside of teen emotions.

Teenagers experience emotions more intensely than adults, both negative and positive. While this can amplify psychological discomfort, it also means that they get more out of pleasures and delights.

Small comforts and joys (like cuddling a pet, being in nature, listening to music, going for a run) are more comforting and joyful to teens than they are for adults. This is why we may find it hard to grasp why watching their favorite movie for the umpteenth time makes a teenager so happy.[3]

I have witnessed this phenomenon repeatedly, and it amazes me how excited teenagers can get over something as minor as chips and queso. Take note of what makes your teenager happy (a day of fly-fishing for your son, fresh chocolate chip cookies for your daughter) and relearn how to love the simple things.

Protect Your Family's Well-Being.

Moms often lose joy when their children struggle. When your child hurts, you hurt, and the pressures that affect your child's joy also affect your joy.

Sadly, today's youth are not in a great place. In record numbers, they're lonely, anxious, depressed, overwhelmed, and burdened by unrealistic expectations. No longer is adolescence an exuberant time of life. Today's teens, for the first time, feel more stressed than their parents.[4]

You can't change the world that is shaping your child, but you can influence the way your child experiences the world. You can be the gatekeeper of their mental health and set goals to reflect your family's idea of success. This may mean choosing a less popular path, like lightening their academic load, but if it inspires more joy for them and your family, then you've made a solid choice.

Limit Your Negative Intake.

What you see, absorb, and take in affects your mood. Whether you're scrolling through social media, watching the news, or spending time with toxic people, it weighs on your spirit.

Did you know anger is the most viral emotion? This explains why many news sources who used to be trustworthy now use salacious headlines and nuclear stories to gain readers and clicks. Gone are the days where journalists had time to prepare stories, check facts, and objectively tell both sides. Now there is a rush to break a story first, even if it means spreading inaccurate news.

Michael Rocque, in *Newsweek,* wrote about social media being a hotbed of false information that often leads to anger. "Collective outrage," he says, "makes us feel good . . . Research has suggested that mob behavior, even violence, can be exciting and 'fun.'"[5]

Negativity dampens joy. And since the human mind gravitates toward negative thoughts, it takes courage and intention to focus on positive thoughts. Now, more than ever, you need positive intakes that feed your soul and spirit.

Move Forward.

Sometimes a lack of joy comes from entering foreign territory. You miss the past and feel nostalgia for what used to be. Especially if your new life is harder, and old comforts are missing, you may yearn for the time when life felt simpler, safer, and happier.

It is normal to feel this way, but dwelling in the past can steal your joy. *To embrace new beginnings, you must let go of your old life.*

God promises to take care of you in Isaiah 43:19 (NLT): "For I am about to do something new. See, I have already begun! Do you not see it? I will make a pathway through the wilderness. I will create rivers in the dry wasteland." Even if your situation appears hopeless, He works miracles. He creates ways to navigate scary new territory. He walks with you and comforts you. He helps you move forward with anticipation.

My friend Annie calls this trust in God "Going Not Knowing." You don't need all the answers because God works out the details. He just wants your obedience in the journey of what will be.

Joy is rooted in hope, and hope is rooted in Jesus. Any pain that you feel today cannot compare to the joy that is coming. While it is tempting to cling to the past, hoping to recapture the greatest joy you have ever known, moving forward is the only option. As J. R. R. Tolkien wrote in *The Hobbit*: "Go back?" he thought. "No good at all! Go sideways? Impossible! Go forward? Only thing to do! On we go!"[6] Even in sorrow, Jesus enters into your heart, uniting you to the source of all joy and peace.

> This is the day the LORD has made. We will rejoice and be glad in it.
>
> PSALM 118:24 (NLT)

PRAY FOR JOY

Joy is more than an emotion. It is also a gift of the Holy Spirit.[7]

Other gifts, known as fruits of the Holy Spirit, are love, peace, forbearance, kindness, goodness, faithfulness, gentleness, and self-control (Galatians 5:22–23).

These gifts help you grow in virtue. They strengthen God's spirit inside you. They fill you up and protect you from the enemy.

In the parable of the empty house in Matthew 12:43–45, Jesus says that an empty house doesn't stay empty. *Something* will fill it up, and without virtue and light inside, darkness and evil will try to come in. Evil will bring its friends too, potentially leaving a person worse off than they were before the impurities were cleaned out of their heart.

So as you fight for joy, you're not just avoiding the black abyss. You're also armoring yourself against a spiritual attack.

Nobody is always joyful. There is a time for sorrow, mourning, grieving, and simply feeling sad. At the same time, joy matters. And if you need mottos that inspire joy, try these:

- It can be hard to find joy around me; that's why I have to find joy within me.
- My joy is rooted in the Lord, not today's circumstances.
- This pain I feel today can't compare to the joy that is coming.
- The Holy Spirit is only a prayer away. It is my lifeline for joy.
- Until God opens the next door, I can praise Him in the hallway.
- I was created for a purpose, and every morning that I wake up means that God has work for me to do.

Where love exists, joy exists. And real joy begins with God's love for you. You can ignore it, but you can't lose it. It is waiting to be found, and as you find it, you give it. You spread the joy that our world needs, joy that awakens the best in humanity and makes you grateful to be alive.

"I have told you this so that my joy may be in you and that your joy may be complete."

JOHN 15:11 (NIV)

What Choosing Joy Models for Your Child

Joyfully, Annie.

That is how I sign my emails. However, my heart isn't always joyful, especially when I'm addressing a difficult issue.

My oldest daughter, Daley, was in her freshman year of college when I knew her joy had been stolen. Moms instinctively sense when worry, doubt, and unworthiness creep in. I call them joy killers. This child was grounded in biblical truth, but the enemy did his best to kill, steal, and destroy her faith foundation. College life was not living up to what she expected, and I was down on my knees. Her joy meter was on empty.

As hard as it is to swallow at times, God wants us to choose joy regardless of the circumstance. James tells us to consider it all joy when we go through trials of many kinds (James 1:2). He never promises it will be easy, but he does promise that choosing joy builds our character and deepens our faith.

Jesus considered joy worthy enough to die for. It was for JOY that Jesus endured the cross (Hebrews 12:1–5). He saw joy in the freedom from sin, belief for all eternity, and the vision of seeing past difficult circumstances to a bigger picture of love.

He chose joy so we can choose joy.

In our house, we have a joy jar. We write down concerns, fears, prayers, and overwhelming situations, and we cast them into the arms of Jesus. We release our joy killers and replace them with trust.

Daley chose to trust. She came home her sophomore year, reaffirmed her faith, and discovered a love for law while working at her father's law firm. She graduated from Auburn University and is currently at Florida State Law School. Her faith is deeper than ever, and her joy meter is full again.

Today, choose joy. Let your children lean on your joy when theirs feels empty. Be aware of the enemy's lies, and keep your eyes on Jesus. Only He can fill your joy meter, and only He can replace your joy killers with deep, abiding trust.

Annie Daley Pajcic
mom of two daughters and two sons

REFLECTION QUESTIONS

1. Have you ever felt joy and sadness on the same day? How did you reconcile the two?

2. "When you wish away the hard parts of a season, you also wish away the good parts." Have you ever regretted wishing away a hard season? Looking back, what would you do differently?

3. Trusting God means trusting in the joy ahead. Name a time when a new situation brought unexpected joy. What did this teach you about God's faithfulness?

4. Are you an optimist or a pessimist? How does a negative environment affect your mood, mindset, and joy?

5. Have you ever seen sadness interrupted by laughter? Share a story about the healing power of laughter.

6. Do you choose joy and fight for it? Do you believe joy is worth fighting for?

6

QUIT THE NEGATIVE SELF-TALK

A Mother Needs to Feel Confident

We have bought the lie that we are victims of our thoughts rather than warriors equipped to fight on the front lines of the greatest battle of our generation: the battle for our minds.

JENNIE ALLEN[1]

Netflix had perfect timing when it released *Tidying Up with Marie Kondo* on New Year's Day.

Like many moms, I kick into declutter-and-purge mode in December. I go through my kids' closets to take inventory of what clothes they have outgrown or no longer wear, and what they might need for Christmas.

And what hits me every December is how we accumulate so much stuff. While I love to organize (and I'm good at organizing), the energy it takes to sift through possessions, determine what is essential, and buy for a family of six can be taxing.

By Christmas Day, I feel spent. And in the weeks leading up to it, I wrestle with guilt. Since I handle all our family's shopping (including gifts from both sides of grandparents), I oscillate between feeling excited by the gifts I find and sickened by the consumerism that gets normalized in our society.

I know the answer is to scale back and give back (and I've done both), yet I'm still hungry for guidance on how to break old habits and make meaningful change.

Enter Marie Kondo, a joyful Japanese decluttering expert and author of the massive hit *The Life-Changing Magic of Tidying Up: The Japanese Art of Decluttering and Organizing*. As I watched her Netflix show, I realized how she appealed to people like me, people living in a country of privilege, yet weighed down by excess.

During the holidays, our problem comes to light, so what better time to shift our habits and thinking than at the start of a new year? Using the KonMari method, Marie Kondo teaches a new way of viewing possessions and keeping a tidy home. You only keep items that "spark joy," and you boldly declutter by using your heart and mind.

While the pros and cons are debatable, KonMari offers a way to live lighter. It gives us permission to let stuff go and be intentional with what we keep. Whether you agree with Marie Kondo or not, she tapped into our desire to simplify. And given her mass appeal (she's been named as one of the 100 Most Influential People by *Time* magazine, and CNN called her book one of the most influential books of the decade),[2] I believe she is living proof that we have an excess problem.

Most of us know that we own too much stuff, and as author Joshua Becker of *Becoming Minimalist* says, we feel the burden. We get a wake-up call from statistics like these:

- The average American home has 300,000 items.
- The average size of the American home has nearly tripled over the past 50 years.
- Despite bigger homes, one out of every ten Americans rent offsite storage—the fastest-growing segment of the commercial real estate industry over the past four decades.
- The average ten-year-old owns 238 toys but plays with just twelve daily.
- Only 3.1 percent of the world's children live in America, but they own 40 percent of the toys consumed globally.
- The average American woman owns thirty outfits. In 1930, that figure was nine.
- The average American throws away sixty-five pounds of clothing per year.
- Women will spend more than eight years of their lives shopping.[3]

In short, we swim in excess. We flock to gurus like Marie Kondo, who help us come up for air and unpack the mess. We have more resources than our ancestors, and that has blurred the lines between "wants" and "needs." We often don't realize we have a problem until we feel the stress of a complicated life.

So how does this relate to negative self-talk? Well, in my opinion, the problem in our minds is a lot like the problem in our homes. Over time, we accumulate mental clutter. We hit a point where we need more head space. The only way to create more head space is to purge unhealthy thoughts and be intentional with what we keep.

Just as we outgrow old clothes, we should also outgrow old mindsets that hinder our personal journey to wellness.

Paul said in 1 Corinthians 13:11 (NIV), "When I was a child, I talked like a child, I thought like a child, I reasoned like a child. When I became a man, I put the ways of childhood behind me." One sign of spiritual maturity and growing in the right direction is breaking old habits and trains of thought that formed when we were young.

We all have negative thought loops and mind scripts that need to go. Yet unlike home clutter, which we can tackle as we see it, we let mental clutter accumulate. We sit with the junk and accept it, forgetting we have the power to choose our thoughts and set our minds free.

Thankfully, our culture now talks about (and values) mental health. We understand the need for healthy thought lives and the impact on wellness. We want a positive life, and since we can't create a positive life while consumed with negative thoughts, we're often forced into a mind edit, a sifting through the mental clutter to kick out negativity.

The expert of a mind edit is God, who created our minds in the first place. He knows our thoughts and offers healthy scripts to replace old ones. His framework is perfect and universally true. Rather than live with mental clutter, we can unpack it and question it. We can free up extra space by eliminating what doesn't belong and incorporating the truths we absolutely need.

> We use God's mighty weapons, not worldly weapons, to knock down the strongholds of human reasoning and to destroy false arguments. We destroy every proud obstacle that keeps people from knowing God. We capture their rebellious thoughts and teach them to obey Christ.
>
> 2 Corinthians 10:4–5 (nlt)

FILTER YOUR THOUGHTS

During parent night at our local junior high, the eighth-grade Advanced English teacher explained his challenging, yet doable, curriculum.

He ended with this:

I want my students to have a love for learning, not a fear of red marks.

As a writer, I wanted to applaud. I've learned firsthand how good editing elevates a writer's work. Once someone points out your mistakes, you don't make those mistakes again. Also, with good editing comes fresh ideas that you'd never think of yourself.

But with my first red-lined manuscript, I got a pit in my stomach. I felt like a massive failure as I scanned the document and saw the red marks jump out. Only when I sat down to read the edits did my attitude shift. My editor's suggestions took the manuscript to the next level. I was thankful the book did not go to print in its original form.

By my third manuscript, I looked forward to edits. Rather than fear red marks, I was curious and ready to learn. By this point I understood how a good editor makes you sound more like yourself; rather than change you, they strengthen your voice.

We all want to be stronger, yet we live in fear of red marks. We look at our lives and despair over all the things that need correction. Rather than approach red marks with curiosity, a chance to grow and improve, we get defensive. We see red marks as signs of massive failure rather than evidence of life in a broken world.

In Alcoholics Anonymous, they have this popular saying: *My mind is a terrible place to be.* The root of many problems is an unhealthy thought life. How you talk to yourself determines how you live, and not processing your life properly can make you feel and act defeated.

As I've said, God created us to live with a spirit of strength, not defeat. He wants our minds to be a healthy escape, a place where truth gets exposed in the light of Christ, not a dark mental prison where shame becomes the bully. Too often, we live in defeat as moms; we inflict red marks on ourselves through negative self-talk.

It may sound like this:

- I'm a terrible mom.
- I'm ruining my kids.
- I've done everything wrong.
- Everyone hates me.
- I'm an idiot.
- I'm a fool.
- I'm just a maid/cook/ chauffeur/bank.
- Nobody cares about me or notices when I'm gone.
- I should stop talking.

- I always say the wrong thing.
- What's the use of trying? Nothing ever changes.
- It all depends on me— and I'm failing.
- I'm not cut out for this.
- I'm not enough.
- I wish I were her.
- How could any man ever want me?
- I'm fat, ugly, and stupid.
- I have no purpose.
- I don't stand a chance.
- My life is over.
- Of course they don't want me.
- We're no longer a family because I got divorced/ my husband left/my husband died.

- It's over for me and my kids.
- What I did is unforgivable. I'm doomed.
- I don't fit in.
- I'll never experience true friendship or find true love.
- God doesn't care about me. I can't remember the last time I felt happy.
- My child is a wreck/my life is a wreck/my house is a wreck.
- I don't deserve joy after what I did.
- It's all my fault.
- My kids deserve better than me.

When we look at ourselves and our lives, the flaws and holes jump out. We get swept up in our thoughts and emotions about what we think is wrong. This makes our minds spin out of control. It fixates our attention on negative assumptions that can become self-fulfilling prophecies.

I'll never forget what a doctor told my mom after a health scare. Suddenly immobile, and with fear in her voice, my mom asked her, "What if I never walk again? What if I'm in a wheelchair the rest of my life?"

The doctor paused and looked my mom straight in the eye.

Slowly and gently, she replied, "Be careful what you wrap your mind around. If you say you'll never walk again, then you'll never walk again."

As a doctor, she understood the power of thoughts. She had seen firsthand how negative thoughts impacted a patient's outcome and mental well-being.

Negative thoughts can sabotage you, and the best way to fight them and develop mature mindsets is to 1) ask God to transform and renew your mind and 2) take your thoughts captive and give them to Christ (Romans 12:2 and 2 Corinthians 10:4–5).

Rather than leave your thinking to chance, or let the world tell you how to think, process your thoughts through the filter of truth.

Jesus brings new life, and thoughts that come from Him are life-giving. They give hope for the future and who you can be. When shame, self-doubt, jealousy, anger, or other hard emotions become the loudest voices in your head, it's time to declutter. It's time to get rid of the mental mess that holds you back.

You can counter negative talk with anchoring thoughts. Imagine how your life might change with these anchors in place:

- God is good. God is love. God loves me.
- I trust God to fill in the gaps of my imperfect life and parenting.
- God is *with* me and *for* me. Even if I lose confidence in myself, I can be confident in Him.
- I'm doing the best I can with a situation that is far from ideal. Even in these circumstances, I can build a great relationship with my child.
- My goal is to keep two feet on the ground. Right now, that is success.
- I'm only human, and humans make mistakes.

- I can only take my children as far as I've come. Becoming a mentally strong mom helps me raise mentally strong kids.
- I'm not an accident. God created me with great intention because the world needs someone exactly like me.
- A healthy thought life deepens my love for Jesus, others, and myself. Thoughts that destroy these relationships aren't from Him.
- I thank God for making me beautiful and giving me the gift of today.
- What people say about me is an opinion. What God says about me is a fact. The way to know my worth is to focus on the facts.
- The Lord is my protector. I have nothing to fear.
- Peace comes when I wrap my mind around truth.
- Not everyone deserves a voice in my life. Not every comment should be taken to heart. I can pray for the wisdom to recognize truth.
- I can survive this devastation. It is temporary, not forever. Better days are ahead.
- I can do all things through Christ who strengthens me.
- My story isn't over. God isn't done with me yet.
- By intentionally choosing my thoughts, I rewrite the scripts in my head.

Negative self-talk robs you of your best life, it spirals into apathy, hopelessness, cynicism, and despair. The enemy will seize any chance to get inside your head, so don't present an open door. Don't ruminate on destructive thoughts.

Protect your mental health, and guard your heart and mind by reflecting on what is true, excellent, praiseworthy, and right (Philippians 4:8). Be a mind warrior, and know that your beliefs set a trajectory for your life. They take you in a positive or negative direction, toward truth or lies, toward hope or uncertainty. Your mindset is your superpower, and when you allow the truth to shape it, you see the world through enlightened eyes.

> Don't copy the behavior and customs of this world, but let God transform you into a new person by changing the way you think. Then you will learn to know God's will for you, which is good and pleasing and perfect.
>
> ROMANS 12:2 (NLT)

REWRITE THE SCRIPTS IN YOUR HEAD

Counselors often talk about the "tapes" in a person's head that play on repeat.

Your tapes are shaped by countless influences, including but not limited to

- your personality;
- your parents;
- your upbringing, family, and sibling dynamics;
- your peers and friends;
- your life experiences and circumstances;
- social media, media, current and past culture; and
- remarks said to you and about you.

Even healthy-minded people have negative scripts, scripts that kick in when you feel insecure, anxious, scared, threatened, depressed, or inadequate. What results is a negative thought loop that turns into negative self-talk.

To stop this talk, you must change your scripts. You need awareness of what you have clung to for years and why your false scripts came about.

Birmingham counselor Julie Sparkman, author of the study *Six Weeks to Sane Thinking* and host of the podcast "Head to Heart: Connect What You Know to How You Live,"[4] says the number-one tape she hears in her office is this:

I'm all alone. If it is to be, it's up to me.

Julie designed her ministry for women who know the truth in their mind but struggle to connect it to their heart. She sees many women who are high performers yet frustrated because they don't get a lot of help, or they think they're incompetent.

One question that Julie helps her clients answer is, "What do you do with the reality of your life . . . especially when it doesn't match the picture in your head that you expected?" How do you respond when life events or people hurt you, disappoint you, or fail to live up to your expectations—or when you disappoint yourself?

Julie says most people have five core tapes, and you can learn your tapes by examining your thoughts for a week and asking someone who knows you to chime in. What are your most recurrent thoughts? What thoughts do you unconsciously resort to? Maybe they sound like this:

Here we go again.
Nothing is better.
I'm the black sheep of my family.
There is something fundamentally wrong with me. I'm incapable.

Whatever your tapes are, there is hope because you can redo your brain's pathways. You can change the way you think *and* the tapes you play. You're not a victim of your mind.

Tremendous research has come out in recent years on neuroplasticity and the brain's remarkable ability to reorganize itself. **Even in adulthood, you can rewire your brain.** You can adapt to new circumstances, learn new things, and be capable of extraordinary change through sustained effort and a healthy lifestyle.[5]

How do you change your self-talk? First, realize that it isn't an overnight fix. It takes work, commitment, and discomfort. Julie Sparkman says we need to increase our tolerance for the unpleasant. This means admitting, identifying, and sitting with difficult thoughts and feelings. The level to which you can sit with your unpleasant thoughts is the level that you can sit with someone else's unpleasant thoughts. As you grow personally, you become better able to help others.

Julie encourages her clients to be aware of what they feel *inwardly* before they respond *outwardly*. Your body sends signals related to the intensity of emotion that you feel (for example, increased heart rate, fast breathing, a tightness in the stomach or chest), and these signals can alert you when you're headed toward an emotional spiral. When intense emotions like panic, confusion, or fury rise up, take the time to regulate them so you don't react out of them.

Also, keep in mind the difference between your amygdala and prefrontal cortex, covered in the anxiety chapter. Your amygdala has three reactions: fight, flight, or freeze.[6] So when you act out of your amygdala, you're driven by survival instincts, not reason. This is crucial during imminent danger, but when your amygdala treats a *perceived* threat like a *real* threat, anxiety spikes and your mind spirals.

The goal is to let your prefrontal cortex, the evolved part of your brain, stay in charge of your self-talk. Rely on your thinking brain, not your emotional brain, and know that when you overreact or feel overly emotional, your amygdala is most likely triggered.

Here are some strategies to cultivate healthy self-talk.

Meditate on Truth.

The best way to retrain your brain is through Christian meditation. To meditate is to think deeply and carefully about something, to focus your mind for spiritual purposes, or to relax.[7]

Choose a Bible verse that speaks to you, and sit with it in a peaceful place. Pray before you start, and ask the Holy Spirit to guide you. Write the verse down, and include surrounding verses for context. Read it multiple times, close your eyes, and reflect on it.

What does God reveal about His character, love, and ways through the verse? How does it apply to your life? What experiences come to mind?

As you reflect on Psalm 9:1 (NLT), for instance ("I will praise you, LORD, with all my heart; I will tell of all the marvelous things you have done"), you may remember an emergency with your son when he fell from a tree and had a brain injury, and God healed him and spared his life. This may lead you to a prayer of thanksgiving, a reminder of God's faithfulness, and a deep conviction to share your story.

Meditation is often misunderstood by Christians because it gets associated with Eastern and new age religions. But unlike Eastern meditation, which advocates emptying the mind, Christian meditation calls us to fill our mind with God and His truth.[8] The Catechism of the Catholic Church says:

Meditation is above all a quest. The mind seeks to understand the why and how of the Christian life, in order to adhere and respond to what the Lord is asking. The required attentiveness is difficult to sustain. We are usually helped by books: the Sacred Scriptures, particularly the Gospels, holy icons, liturgical texts of the day or season, writings of the spiritual fathers, works of spirituality, the great book of creation, and that of history, the page on which the "today" of God is written . . . the important thing is to advance, with the Holy Spirit, along the one way of prayer: Christ Jesus.[9]

Meditating on truth is a form of prayer. It helps you hear, listen, and unite with God.

Think for Yourself.

We live in an age of mob mentality, herd mentality, and groupthink. A world where people set aside their personal beliefs to adopt the beliefs of a group.

Letting other people think for you puts you at the mercy of their motives, moods, values, experiences, and humanity. Even the smartest people aren't always right, and joining every angry bandwagon will eventually make you an angry person.

Rather than blindly accepting groupthink, wait for the truth to emerge. Do your research, dig deep before forming an opinion, and know that you can consider a thought without accepting it.

Spend Time with Healthy-Minded People.

There is an old saying that if you spend enough time at the barber shop you'll eventually get a haircut. The company you keep rubs off, influencing your thoughts, choices, mindsets, and actions.

It brings out the *best* or the *worst* in you.

Be kind but create boundaries with negative people. Don't give them a voice in your life or a megaphone to critique you. Some people aren't good for you. They don't want you to succeed or outdo them. It is better to walk away than to allow them to shape your thought life.

When deciding who to include in your most trusted circle, ask yourself these questions:

- Would I act on their advice?
- Do I respect them and admire their character?
- Do they love me and see the good?
- Do I feel uplifted after being with them?
- Do they inspire my faith and help me feel closer to the people who love me most, like my family?
- Do they genuinely care about me?
- Do their choices produce good fruit in their life, like healthy relationships?

If you answered *no*, then reconsider your circle. Turn your attention toward healthy-minded people.

Expect Life to Be Hard.

We assume that life should always be easy. When it's not, we assume we're doing it wrong.

But on any path, there will be problems. And if you expect a smooth ride, you'll end up disillusioned, angry, or bitter. A better option is to expect challenges and know that God is always available to help. Trials are inevitable, but the attitude you bring into your trials will influence the outcome and shape your self-talk.

Know Yourself.

Growth requires self-awareness. By identifying triggers that undo you, you can interrupt unhealthy thoughts.

It's possible to feel like a failure all day as events like these unfold:

- You walk into your teenager's room and are disgusted by the mess.
- You're late picking up your son from practice, and he is the only child left.
- You take your preschooler to Target, and she pitches a tantrum on the floor.
- You glance in the laundry room, and the monstrous pile taunts you.
- You check your child's grades and see a D on their latest test.
- You get a phone call and hear that your child made a big mistake.
- You check social media and realize you were excluded from a girls' night.
- You put on your favorite jeans and feel your recent weight gain.

Add these up, and you have the makings of a pity party. Tack on other events (being ignored by other moms, hanging up on your mom, snapping at your best friend, screaming at your family, getting passed over for a promotion, crying when nothing is wrong) and your self-talk can go ballistic.

Sometimes the real problem runs deeper than the surface. Maybe it crushes you to be ignored because you're insecure about your friendships. Maybe you're mad at your mom because she triggers your guilt. Maybe you lash out at your family because you fear that nobody loves you as much as you love them. Maybe losing the promotion makes you feel undervalued. Maybe you cry because you're lonely.

In these moments, press the reset button. Be gentle with yourself ,and stop dwelling on a sense of failure.

Work Through Your Resentments Daily.

Nothing ruins a beautiful mind like resentment. Resentment stems from past hurts and, left unchecked, will manifest as ill will, pride, anger, bitterness, grudges, jealousy, and a refusal to forgive.

Harboring resentment makes you sick. It is often described as drinking poison and expecting the other person to die; it hurts *you* more than *them.* Anything that hardens your heart also hardens you to God's spirit. Forgiveness matters; without it, you stay stuck.

My friend in addiction recovery told me how they start each day with gratitude and end each day by working through that day's resentments. Whether you resent your boss, your family, your church, or something else, the goal is to take accountability for your role in each conflict and process little grudges and disappointments so they don't become big grudges and disappointments.

Have a Mental Battle Plan.

I once sat next to a woman on an airplane who spent years in a mentally abusive marriage. While she is thriving now, it took her years to renew her mindset—and help from a neighbor who boosted her confidence.

One way she rebuilt her life was by finding Scripture to counter her husband's remarks. When he told her, "You're such a burden!" she'd tell herself, "Carry each other's burdens." She also kept a Bible on her bedstand, because as her neighbor pointed out, friends and family aren't always available to talk at 2:00 a.m., but Jesus is.

The enemy is real, and as I discuss in the Fight the Good Fight chapter, he requires a mental battle.

Aligning your thoughts with God's thoughts won't happen automatically. It takes prayer, intention, and determination. From the stories you tell yourself to the lies of Satan and our culture, there are forces at work that can mess with your mind and your confidence.

Thankfully, God is greater. The Spirit who lives in you is greater than the spirit who lives in the world. Even a quick prayer like "Help me, Jesus!" can open the door to new insight and protection.

Shift Your Perspective.

In any situation, there are multiple perspectives available. The goal is to look through God's lens.

He is a God of compassion and second chances. He meets you where you are, yet he doesn't leave you there. Even when your self-talk goes ballistic, you can shift to this perspective:

Rather than beat myself up, I'll set a good example. I'll let my kids witness my brave steps to get us to a better place. They'll see me trust God and credit Him as my source of strength. They'll learn lessons as they watch me persevere. They won't be disillusioned when they face their own battles; in some ways, they'll be prepared.

I can share my mistakes as a cautionary tale. I can teach my children that life isn't fair, and sometimes we suffer because of other people's choices or unforeseen events. I can teach my sons to respect women and inspire my daughters to be strong women. After watching my sacrifices, they may understand how fiercely I love them . . . if not now, then one day.

Studies show that many resilient adults experienced trauma as children. Dr. Michele Borba, in her brilliantly researched book *Thrivers: The Surprising Reasons Why Some Kids Struggle and Others Shine,* says that one commonality among Thrivers is that they have caring adults in their corner who offer hope.[10] Let this motivate you to build a healthy thought life. Even in traumatic times, you can be that hopeful adult for your kids.

In Summary, the Scripts in Your Head Are Malleable. And once you know better, you can think better. Even if you've operated by unhealthy scripts in the past, you can choose new scripts today, bringing clarity into your mind and optimism into your future.

> Set your minds on things above, not on earthly things.
> Colossians 3:2 (NIV)

BUILD YOUR MENTAL ARMOR

Cleaning out your mental closet is a lifelong process. Nobody ever "arrives" and wakes up in this life with a suddenly pristine mind.

Even as you discard and replace old mindsets, triggers can take you back to old patterns of thinking. Around your family, for instance, you may become that twelve-year-old girl who

- feels like her voice isn't heard;
- believes her brother is her father's favorite;

- tries to please her mom, yet always feels like a disappointment;
- had so many problems growing up that nobody sees her success as an adult;
- engages in immature fights because the family dynamic from childhood never evolved;
- feels helpless against a domineering relative; or
- feels different than the group, not accepted or understood.

When an old mindset sneaks up on you, bring it to light. Ask, "How can I break this cycle? How can I choose a better mindset? How can I protect my mental health?"

You can't control anyone else's thoughts, but you *can* control your own. You can build mental resilience and fortitude. *Notice what goes through your mind, and be selective about what you keep.* It's never too late to change your mind or adopt a healthier train of thought.

Just as your body grows up and matures, your mindsets should mature too. Outgrow old patterns that hold you back, and adopt new thoughts that reflect God's love and desire for your ultimate good.

> You will keep in perfect peace all who trust in you, all whose thoughts are fixed on you!
>
> ISAIAH 26:3 (NLT)

What Healthy Self-Talk Models for Your Child

Years ago, my oldest child experienced a difficult time at school.

My child who loved school started to dread it, and when I was with him, I stayed positive. But when I wasn't with him, negative thoughts crept in. *What haven't I taught him? What could I have done to prevent his pain?* In an attempt to gain control, my thoughts were focused on myself, not my son.

Clarity seemed miles away as I struggled to discern whether this was a growth experience or something bigger where I should intervene. I didn't want to be "that mom" or jump in too quickly. I prayed hard for guidance.

Tough days followed, and as his situation escalated, I discovered my youngest child was struggling too. Her situation was even worse, which really fueled the negative thoughts. *Have I done everything I can do for my children? Why are both of them struggling?*

The irony is, I'm a psychologist. I'm an expert at picking up subtleties of behavior. But with my own children, my expert training and objectivity appeared useless. Blind spots existed, and negative loops gained momentum by the day.

At work, I had several big projects planned. And at home, my children needed more time and attention. As the tension between home and work heightened, I slowly gained clarity and knew what I had to do.

One, I needed to alter my work schedule, keeping hours at a bare minimum and putting projects on hold. Two, I needed space—space to process my thoughts, figure out next steps, and save my energy. My mantra became **Grace and Space.** When negative thoughts surfaced, I practiced grace and self-compassion. I sought counsel from a friend and asked God to use our situation for good.

Over time, more clarity came—doors opened, and we made some tough decisions.

Today, both my children are thriving. One recently won a character award at school. When this child told me, "My experience made me realize that I never want another person to feel the way I did," I smiled. God led us down the path to His plan.

In my practice, I see moms struggle all the time with the same negative loops. We can be so hard on ourselves and easily lose our energy and focus. Trusting God, giving ourselves grace and space, and building in time for self-care and reflection are essential tools we need. They are also life skills our children need when negative loops get the best of them.

Dr. Rachel Blake Fry
mom of one son and one daughter

REFLECTION QUESTIONS

1. On a scale of one to ten, how much mental clutter do you have? Explain.

2. Identify five core scripts that play in your head. Which one is most dominant?

3. Replace one old thought pattern with one new thought pattern. How does this mind shift affect your confidence, motivation, or hope?

4. How do you respond to negative thoughts? Do you fight them, believe them, dwell on them, or compare them to God's Word to see if they're true?

5. One sign of spiritual maturity is breaking old habits and trains of thought that formed when we were young. What childhood script can you outgrow to become a healthy-minded adult?

6. Have negative thought loops ever clouded your clarity? If so, how did you regain clarity?

7

MAKE PEACE WITH YOUR BODY

A Mother Needs to Feel Beautiful

*You all can judge my body all you want, but
at the end of the day it's MY body. I love
it and I'm comfortable in my own skin.*

Simone Biles[1]

I was a junior in high school when my friend suggested that we make ourselves regurgitate our food.

We were at a sleepover, and we had just gorged on everything from Cool Ranch Doritos to cookie cake. We had that sick, gluttonous, regretful feeling of indulging in too much at once. This seemed like an easy solution.

To be honest, purging what I had eaten had never crossed my mind, but you know how they say that teenagers are vulnerable to the power of suggestion? Well, this was a prime example. We didn't want our feast to go to our hips, and in some weird, twisted way, this sneaky rebellion in our friend's bathroom triggered the adrenaline rush that teenagers crave.

I wasn't successful that night, but in the months to come I learned how to do it. I also learned how to starve myself, which opened a new door to weight management.

The timing worked because I'd gained a few pounds after I quit cheerleading. I was studying more and exercising less, and the junk food habits I got away with as an athlete caught up with me. Although my appearance looked largely the same (one perk of being 5'8" is that extra pounds have room to spread out), I knew the difference. I wanted my athletic body back.

The summer before my senior year, my regimen amped up. Like many girls, I embarked on a quest to make my senior year the best year yet, and because I am disciplined and goal-oriented, I spent that summer attaining a savage tan and achieving a record-low weight. While some people commented that I looked too thin, I took it as a badge of honor and felt good about the track I was on.

What happened inside me, I now realize, was also happening around me. *Other girls were shrinking too, and each one garnered positive attention and praise.* From what I could see, the biggest reaction came from girls, not guys. With each body transformation, girls were the ones who acted obsessed.

The biggest buzz in school (and most drastic makeover) happened to a girl in our extended friend group. She turned a new leaf as she morphed into a super-fit aerobics instructor. At first, she looked amazing, but as her weight fell to dangerous levels, she sought treatment. Soon after, her close friend told us this: "Her mom said that we need to stop complimenting her. According to her therapist, all the praise she hears at school fuels her motivation to keep losing weight. We are making it worse."

It never occurred to me that we, her friends, could be part of the problem. And although I didn't want to end up in treatment too, I continued with my unhealthy habits. With prom, senior events, and college around the corner, I wanted to look as impressive and perfect as possible.

For our senior trip we took a cruise and I got sick. I felt horrible and spent most of the trip sleeping. The ship's doctor diagnosed me with the worst case of tonsillitis he'd ever seen, but it wasn't until days later, when I got off the bus at pickup and fell limply into my parents' arms, that the severity of my health issue kicked in.

My parents took me straight to an emergency clinic, where we learned that I had a fever of 104 degrees and mononucleosis. I spent the next two months at home with my mom nursing me back to health. She later told me that watching me get off that bus was one of her most frightening moments as a parent. She had no idea I was even sick because the chaperones for our senior trip didn't tell her.

You would think that experience might teach me a lesson,

that I'd put two and two together and understand how a lack of proper nutrition made me weak and vulnerable to illness, but college brought new issues. I was surrounded by gorgeous girls, constantly going to parties, and eating pizza at midnight.

Starving myself felt impossible with junk food so readily available, and by October I had gained the notorious Freshman Fifteen. I hated how I looked, and though I did pick up one new healthy habit, exercising with friends, I still wasn't eating well.

Living in a dorm took purging off the table, but one day, after binging on my roommate's leftover pizza while she was gone, I felt desperate. Not wanting to use the community bathroom, I found a paper bag and got sick in it.

That was my rock-bottom moment. I was so grossed out and mad at myself that I finally felt the motivation to find a healthier way and quit sabotaging myself.

Slowly, over time, I built healthier habits with food and exercise. I still had issues to work through, however, and over the years I've been guilty of all the common mistakes that females make: overexercising, undereating, overeating, hating my body, obsessing over my body, and giving too much time, attention, and mind space to my physical appearance.

Having four daughters has forced me to deal with my baggage. *It has made me think long and hard about the example I hope to set for them and what I need to work on.* While I'm not in a perfect place, I have come a *long* way since that night in my friend's bathroom. I now have these advantages working in my favor:

- More self-awareness and self-compassion
- A better understanding of nutrition and health
- Better health goals and stronger convictions
- A desire for long-term wellness

- Awareness of the enemy's lies and how they mess with my self-esteem
- A deep understanding of God's truth
- Gratitude for what my body can do
- Motivation to find balance in not paying too *much* attention or too *little* attention to the one body I have
- Children who inspire me to grow a healthy relationship with my body and with food

I share all of this to clarify how I am a work in progress. Part of my wellness journey is learning how to love, take care of, and make peace with my own body. As women, we often make great strides in our thirties and forties, finally accepting ourselves and feeling comfortable in our skin, yet as we push fifty (where our bodies change again and looks begin to notably decline), old insecurities can crop up. It doesn't help as we scroll through social media and compare ourselves to women much younger than us.

We live in a world that worships beauty and lavishes praise as our bodies shrink. We gain attention as our beauty peaks and lose attention as it fades. In this culture, where females are expected to be flawless, it is easy to be consumed by pursuits that steal our contentment and joy.

None of us have the dewy charm of youth, but we *do* have experience. We've seen how a woman's body can grow and birth babies, comfort and nurture loved ones, and handle huge life demands (among other miracles). Comparing these purposes to looking hot in a bikini makes the latter goal look trite. *Everything God makes is good, and since He made our bodies, they are good too.* He helps us love and accept ourselves. He loves us in every shape and season.

My body-image issues arose because I didn't know better. *I was young, naïve, and gullible, the product of an uneducated generation and a fallen world.* I share my mistakes with my daughters and others as a cautionary tale. My hope for every female is that we grow daily in our awareness of this: a girl's best asset is her soul, and the purpose of her body is to protect that soul and put it into motion.

> Do you not know that your bodies are temples of the Holy Spirit, who is in you, whom you have received from God? You are not your own; you were bought at a price. Therefore honor God with your bodies.
>
> 1 CORINTHIANS 6:19–20 (NIV)

BE GOOD TO YOUR BODY

Across the world today, the wellness industry is booming.

More than ever, people want to take charge of their health. They want to prevent illness, not just treat it. They want healthy lifestyle habits that help them become their best self physically, mentally, and emotionally.

Attention to wellness is good, but in many cases it has created a fixation on healthy living. It has led to surging consumer demand in an already lucrative industry. As a result, we get inundated every day with health, fitness, and nutrition advice. From social media influencers to wellness coaches and nutritionists, people have come out of the woodwork to help us live our best lives.

While some coaches are trained, some are not. What often results is viral misinformation and misguided gurus who demonize food, create a toxic diet culture, or contribute to a rapidly growing problem called orthorexia.

Orthorexia is an unhealthy obsession with eating only "clean" or "pure" food. Propelled by the clean food movement (started by consumers who demand ingredient transparency and knowing what goes into their bodies), orthorexia is overly rigid and strict.

At first the goal is innocent—to eat healthier. But as the diet gets more restrictive, malnourishment occurs. Someone with orthorexia may eliminate processed foods, then meat, then dairy, then carbs, and so on until they get down to ten or fewer foods they allow themselves to eat. Since their diet appears healthy, orthorexia can fly under the radar. *It has less stigma than traditional eating disorders and hides under the guise of "good health."*

As a mom with kids who have food allergies, I'm thankful for the clean food movement. It helps me keep my kids safe and monitor their food. I'm also glad that I can make informed decisions. Today's parents are wellness-minded because we have more information. We are aware of what's good for our bodies.

Personally, I expect our golden years to be more golden than our parents' generation because we know that eating well, exercising, and building positive health habits now improve our odds later. We have science and research teaching us about gut health, brain foods, probiotics, and holistic wellness. We understand the mind-body-soul connection and the impact of food and exercise on our mental health and risk of disease.

Our parents, on the other hand, probably never considered how much sugar was in a Coke or what eating bacon every day might do to their arteries. They weren't encouraged to exercise unless they were athletes. Even smoking was different; many of them got hooked before the hazards were publicly known. When it came to their health, they made less-informed decisions.

The world shaping us is vastly different. We live in a time where terms like keto, Whole30, digestive harmony, hydration, meditation, healthy fats, healthy carbs, plant-based foods, processed food, organic, meals that heal, kombucha, collagen powder, Peloton, and SoulCycle are part of the culture. Yet with each new trend or advancement, new issues arise.

While it is wonderful that we take charge of our health, we've also seen wellness become an idol. God's goal is to make us heaven-ready, not magazine-ready, and some pursuits that we chase in the name of "wellness" can distract us from building a healthy self-image. They can make us prioritize outer beauty over inner beauty.

So how do you give your body the attention it deserves without creating an idol? How do you avoid excess or extremes and work toward balanced health?

I believe the best guiding forces are *God* and *moderation.* I believe the healthiest people eat balanced meals, practice portion control, and move a lot. They don't let food control their life or dwell in guilt when they slip. Rather than expect perfection, they eat within a 90/10 or 80/20 ratio of whole foods/moderate splurges. They choose foods that make them feel good while leaving room for treats.

Rather than demonize pizza (or make it the forbidden fruit), they see a food that is less healthy than other options, but one they can occasionally enjoy in small portions, if they choose, to avoid binging later.

Making peace with your body is a personal journey, and only you can decide what works best for you. Finding healthy ways to be healthy keeps you from becoming a slave to food or your body.

Ultimately, a healthy body begins with a healthy mind. Here are eight mindsets to inspire better body love:

1. See food as fuel.

The fact is, food gives you energy. Treating it as a necessity, not temptation, inspires a healthy relationship.

Seventy-five percent of Americans have an unhealthy relationship with food.[2] More than 30 million people in America suffer from an eating disorder—and even more deal with disordered eating symptoms.[3]

Disordered eating, where habits become rigid or compulsive, often precedes eating disorders. The problem can snowball because it is less likely to be caught and treated early. Consider these facts too:

- Middle-age women are the fastest-growing segment of the population being diagnosed with eating disorders.
- One in five women struggle with an eating disorder or disordered eating.
- Americans spend over $40 billion on dieting and diet-related products each year.[4]

It is a wake-up call to hear that eating disorders and body dissatisfaction among older populations are on the rise. With more women over fifty engaging in disordered eating (from creating rules to obsessing over being thin), we have proof that this can be a lifelong struggle.

A healthy diet is more essential with age because your need for vitamins and minerals increases after age fifty. Regular exercise and proper nutrition help prevent a variety of ailments.[5] There are many food philosophies, but I believe the best ones reflect the Mediterranean diet, which has a long history of success.

You and I both need food to survive. Your intake affects your health, sleep, moods, hormones, sex drive, brain, energy, and emotions. Consider how different foods make you feel, listen to your body, and choose foods that help you operate at peak capacity.

2. Search for purpose.

Mother Teresa once referred to herself as "a pencil in God's hand." She knew that her work was made possible only by His power inside her.[6]

The same is true for you. Your body is God's tool, an instrument of His love and peace. Your purpose is far bigger than physical perfection.

If your friend needs a hug or dinner delivered to her doorstep, God uses you to do it. If your son needs advice or your daughter needs encouragement, God uses you to speak it out loud. Every day, He accomplishes good work through you. He moves through you, speaks through you, and shines light through you.

Focusing on what your body *does* keeps you from fixating on how it *looks.* Obsessing over your appearance won't make anyone a better person, but what does add value to the lives around you is living out your purpose.

Reflect on your strengths and capabilities, and let your body be God's pencil.

3. Understand cultural influences.

America's obsession with thinness began in the 1960s, when super-skinny models such as Twiggy became the new epitome of beauty.

Some experts trace the rise in anorexia back to this significant shift in ideal body shapes. **Models with waif-like frames marked a big departure from traditional ideals of beauty, embodied by voluptuous figures like Marilyn Monroe.** From the late 1960s onward, female models and celebrities continued to shrink.[7]

Today, this thin ideal gets fueled by social media, airbrushed models, and a beauty industry that profits from our animosity toward the mirror. When Cindy Crawford famously said, "Even I don't wake up looking like Cindy Crawford,"[8] she validated what we all know deep down: beauty is never as effortless or as honest as advertisers want us to believe. They make money by promising their products will solve all of our problems.

Our culture loves to sow discontent, because making us feel physically inadequate keeps the beauty industry in business. You, however, get to choose what sinks in. You decide how far you'll go to achieve beauty ideals.

4. Cultivate inner beauty.

Looks are a depreciating asset, and the older you get, the more your inner beauty matters.

How you act (and make people feel) impacts the way people see you. Beauty is a running tally influenced by a woman's choices, and many outwardly beautiful females make themselves ugly by acting catty, vindictive, or mean. They start as a ten on the beauty scale and fall to a seven as their true colors show.

Then there are females with so much character and inner light that they rise from a seven to a ten. Once you know them, a deeper beauty shines through: God's presence inside of them.

Your beauty quotient grows by simply being kind. And you can feel more attractive by using your heart, brain, and talent, all of which can appreciate and get better with time. Appearance is a starting point, and what makes people crave your company runs deeper than the eye can see.

5. Remember, young eyes are watching.

Our body issues hurt us as moms. They also hurt our children. Those of us with daughters are especially mindful of this. Research consistently shows that the same-sex parent is the most important role model for a child—and the greatest influence on a girl's body image is her mom.

"Even if a mom says to the daughter, 'You look so beautiful, but I'm so fat,' it can be detrimental," says Dr. Leslie Sim, clinical director of Mayo Clinic's eating disorders program.[9] A poor body image is often passed on from one generation to another.

An obsession with health does damage as well. *As my daughter recently told me, most girls on TikTok who discuss their eating disorders talk about their overly healthy moms.* Watching their mothers exercise two hours a day (and live on lettuce, tomatoes, and barely enough food) compelled them to do the same. Even when we think we're setting a good example, we can send the wrong message.

The good news is, we can break unhealthy cycles. We can make friends with our mirror and stop the abuse. Our children need healthy influences because they're surrounded by unhealthy ones. They're growing up in an age of thinspiration websites that glamorize anorexia, promote crash diets, and give advice on how to suppress hunger, induce vomiting, and skip meals without their family noticing.

What once got shared among girlfriends is now available on the Internet. Simply Google "Pro-Ana" or "Pro-Mia" (short for Pro-Anorexia and Pro-Bulimia) and you'll find meeting places that encourage girls in all the wrong ways.

Loving your body has wide implications, impacting you and the next generation. Even your son is influenced by your attitude toward your body, and if all he hears is criticism, he may project impossible expectations onto his future wife.

6. Choose new scripts.

In the self-talk chapter, I discussed mental scripts. You probably have a negative body script (or two) that needs to be replaced.

As you create new scripts, remember the following:

- *Emotion follows motion.* Acting lovingly toward yourself (even if you don't feel it yet) and saying loving remarks (even if you don't believe them yet) point you down the right path. Simple affirmations like *I love the strong legs that let me run* can get you started.
- *The enemy wants you to stop serving God.* What better ploy than to mess with your confidence or make you self-consumed? When self-hatred or self-focus cloud your focus, Satan may be at work.
- *You are made in God's image. Even as your body changes, His love doesn't.* As you look in the mirror, notice what you love—your periwinkle eyes, your easy smile, the dimples in your cheeks—and give thanks for your uniqueness.
- *Habits are best changed one at a time.* If you've neglected your body, take small steps forward. Overcome one hurdle at a time. Spend one week choosing healthy breakfast options, another week perusing the grocery store with an eye on wellness, and another week learning from a trainer or a coach. Breaking down your plan into doable goals helps you feel capable and accomplished.
- *You can love your body even as you improve your habits.* My friend who is a certified eating disorder specialist told me about a Peloton instructor who always talks about how your body is a masterpiece *and* a work in progress. She loves this mindset of embracing your body as God's masterpiece, even as it changes.
- *Meals build community.* Rather than fixate on your food, focus on the people you share meals with. Get lost in great conversations that help you quit overthinking what you should or shouldn't eat.
- *Being a slave to your body, your makeup, or your mirror is no way to live.* Whatever it takes, break the chain.

- *No woman is meant to look like a human x-ray.* Contrary to current trends, a healthy amount of body fat is essential for your survival, immunity, hormones, and proper body function.
- *Healthy people seek help.* There is no shame in reaching out when you feel out of your league. If anything, it shows self-love and self-awareness. I know many wonderful counselors who specialize in body image, and any therapy that helps you reclaim your life is worth the cost.

What you tell yourself matters, and what you play on repeat matters more. Replace body scripts that you've outgrown with scripts that show maturity.

7. Aim to feel good.

Health isn't about your size; it's about feeling good so you can handle your life. The following basics can boost your well-being

- drinking water
- stretching
- providing your body with proper nutrition
- engaging in physical activity
- releasing stress through exercise
- sleep
- getting out of bad relationships
- monitoring your mental health
- showing grace (to yourself and others)
- limiting technology
- setting boundaries
- expressing your needs
- leaving room for rest and fun
- protecting your spiritual health

Think about the things that give you life or energy (making your favorite smoothie, talking to a therapist, getting dressed every day, taking a Pilates class), and carve out time and resources to make them happen. Only you know what makes you feel good.

8. Expect body changes.

Your body evolves over time. It won't always do what it once did. Even if you stay in amazing shape, you can't compete with your younger self.

I noticed a difference in my body, for instance, between my first child and last child. I delivered Ella at age thirty and Camille at thirty-seven. With Ella I bounced back fast, yet Camille was harder. I was seven years older and felt my age.

In every season, your body is good. It is worthy of care and respect. Rather than compare yourself to the young moms pushing strollers, or to celebrities with trainers and chefs, take pride in where you are. Eat well and work out because you love your body, not because you hate it. Avoid unhealthy extremes, seek balance, and know that like most things in life, your body is always subject to change.

At any age, hearing praise about your body can be addictive. It can keep you seeking human approval at the expense of your health.

A physical transformation may bring applause, but a mental transformation is what brings you peace. *Don't discount your mental victories. Don't discredit the progress that no one sees.* What happens inside you impacts the world around you, and as you grow healthy from the inside out, you reap rewards that money can't buy.

The most beautiful women are first and foremost beautiful souls. Nurture your body so your soul can shine, and treat your body as worthy of praise, because it is.

> For everything created by God is good, and nothing is to be rejected if it is received with thanksgiving, for it is made holy by the word of God and prayer.
>
> 1 TIMOTHY 4:4–5 (ESV)

THINK LONG TERM

As my daughters became teenagers, I amped up the talks about alcohol, vaping, drugs, and harmful substances.

I reiterated this point:

> You only get *one* body in life, and it has to last you a long time (possibly eighty or ninety years), so be good to it. Make healthy choices and think twice before putting anything potentially harmful in your body. Choices that seem harmless now, choices your classmates will make in the years ahead, can set you up for lifelong problems. They can cause serious issues that you wouldn't wish on your worst enemy.

I'd then illustrate with stories, like the story about the pulmonologist who told my friend how he is seeing a new category of patients: young people in their twenties who will need lung transplants one day because vaping has ruined their lungs.

I'd talk about how many people my age struggle with alcoholism and, in some cases, have lost everything they care about—their spouse, their kids, and their job—because addiction is incredibly hard to overcome. Research shows that the earlier a person starts drinking, the more prone they are to addiction.

Finally, I'd talk about the research that has emerged regarding the teenage brain, how making poor choices while your brain is still developing (and rapidly firing synapses) can set up harmful pathways that cost you your future hopes and dreams.

In short, I centered these conversations around *health*. I reminded my girls to protect their health in body, mind, and spirit. At age sixteen and sixty, our choices have consequences for our future. Maturity helps us see the link.

One way to make peace with your body is to think about the future. Ask yourself, "Where do I hope to be in thirty years, and what choices should I make today to get there?"

Personally, I hope for a lifetime of active living. I want to be a healthy, energetic grandparent. I want to watch my kids and grandkids grow up. I want to support and encourage my daughters in their busy adult lives.

This vision propels me. It inspires me to take care of my body, pray for good health, and not make dumb choices like I did as a teenager based on short-term gratification.

I often remind myself that when we die, our earthly bodies die too. We could spend decades sculpting a masterpiece of flesh that is rendered worthless the moment we pass. At our funerals, nobody will be talking about our six-pack abs or the size of our thigh gap. What people will talk about is the kind of person we were, our impact on them, and how we created a better world.

We live in a culture that begins teaching us in childhood to critique, dissect, and perfect our bodies. It judges us based on impossibly high ideals. It can take a lifetime to unwire these mindsets and listen instead to the inner voice that speaks kindly to our imperfect selves.

The best part of you (or anyone) isn't readily apparent. Even if you won the genetic lottery, this is true. *It is your soul, not your body, that is your ticket to heaven, so look past the eye's approval when practicing body positivity.* Give thanks for the body you have and the life it allows you to live as you journey through this earth.

> But the LORD said to Samuel, "Do not consider his appearance or his height, for I have rejected him. The LORD does not look at the things people look at. People look at the outward appearance, but the LORD looks at the heart."
>
> 1 SAMUEL 16:7 (NIV)

What Making Peace with Your Body Models for Your Child

My first diet started at age nineteen when the enemy whispered the lie, "You don't look like a personal trainer." Even though I was healthy and not overweight—and had plenty of clients—this lie spiraled into an eating disorder where I was terrified of looking fat. All the compliments inspired me to overexercise and undereat, and though I knew I had gotten too thin, I felt stuck.

Before long I gave myself "cheat days." I drove my starving body from bakery to bakery and ate until I got sick, assuring myself that the diet would start tomorrow. Again, I felt stuck, trapped in the bondage of an all-or-nothing, restrict-binge cycle.

Getting married and having children put me in a better place because I was happy. Still, I wanted to be healthier, so I did Whole30. I loved how I felt and decided to be paleo. But as a pizza night or celebrating with birthday cake started to make me feel guilty, I felt my old bondage creep back in. The Lord convicted me, helping me see how my desire to be "healthy" consumed my daily thoughts.

Today, I have found peace with my body and food. I live in a gray area instead of the black-and-white mindset of "good foods" and "bad foods" and overthinking every bite. The Lord has turned my passion into a business where I now coach women and teens to properly feed and move their bodies to a place of abundance and freedom. It is possible, and what I hope to model for my children and clients is the positive impact we can have as we free up the brain space we've wasted on unhealthy obsessions with body image, food, or exercise and use it instead to help others.

Meredith Grant Mann
founder of The Peachie Spoon and mom of two sons
and one daughter

REFLECTION QUESTIONS

1. What was your relationship with food and your body as a teenager? What would you tell your teenage self now?

2. Do you believe wellness, taken to an extreme, can be an idol? Why or why not?

3. When choosing foods, do you let moderation be your guide? Are you more prone to undereat or overeat? Share your story.

4. Throughout your life, your body and hormone levels change. What recent changes have you wrestled with? What has helped you to move (or prevented you from moving) forward?

5. Where do you hope to be in thirty years? What healthy body choices can you make today to get there?

6. Has a desire to be "healthy" ever consumed your thoughts? Have you ever fallen into an unhealthy obsession with body image, food, or exercise? Moving forward, how can you find freedom?

8

FIGHT THE GOOD FIGHT

A Mother Needs to Feel Capable

*I am not afraid of opposition. My
God is a God of battles.*

G. K. CHESTERTON[1]

I met her in a self-defense class, a grown woman the size of a fifth-grader.

I didn't even notice her standing beside me in the circle. I had signed up for this class with my daughter and her friends, and honestly, she blended in with the seventh-grade girls. She had to weigh less than a hundred pounds, and I would soon find out why.

"I'm going through a terrible divorce," she whispered, her voice shaky and faint. "My husband has been awful, and I have no confidence left. That's why I'm taking this class, to feel better about myself. To build my self-esteem."

My heart went out to this sweet woman. I felt compassion and admiration for her courage. She looked like she had hit rock bottom, yet she was fighting to get back on her feet: fighting for her kids, herself, and her job. I was surprised to learn she was a doctor, and I realized then how even the highest education couldn't protect her mind from a mentally abusive marriage.

I connected her with a friend who had overcome a similar situation. We emailed a few times, and I didn't see her again until two years later, when we crossed paths at our kids' middle school. She reintroduced herself, and I was glad she did, because I never would have recognized her.

She was still small, only now she was lean and healthy, having gained some weight and muscle.

She smiled brightly and spoke confidently.

She had on a flattering outfit, not baggy clothes.

And, most notably, she was glowing. *She had the light back in her eyes, a light that was missing the first time I met her.*

"My ex-husband is still terrible to me," she told me matter-of-factly, "but I'm in a much better place than the last time you saw me. I've learned how to handle him."

I couldn't believe her transformation, and I was so happy for her. I walked away feeling inspired by what I learned from this woman.

One, when she took that self-defense class, she was not in fighting condition physically or mentally, yet she did it anyway. She didn't wait until she felt "ready."

Two, she showed up alone and didn't worry about what others might think.

Three, she was internally broken, yet she knew that empowering herself physically would boost her confidence mentally. There is a deep connection between the mind, body, and soul—and progress in one area strengthens the other areas.

Four, she was hardly eating when I met her, and she knew she was headed for trouble. Rather than resign herself to that path, she chose better. She practiced the self-care that is essential to recovery.

Five, her circumstances had not changed, but *she* had changed, and this equipped her to take back the power that her ex-husband used to diminish her.

And six, she began with baby steps. She understood how courage means stepping forward even when you are scared or fragile. It means trying a crazy idea (like a self-defense class) that may lead to answers. It means redefining "strength" and showing the heart of a warrior even when your face doesn't look like a warrior.

Your trials in life may not be this extreme, but you will face challenges that shape you, test you, and push you toward a breaking point. Life isn't hard because you do it all wrong; it's hard because you want to do it right. *We live in a broken world, yet our real home is in heaven, and until God restores this world and claims a final victory, we will fight a battle of good versus evil.*

If you're awake to the truth, then you'll feel this battle. You'll know how difficult it is to choose what is right over what is easy or popular. G. K. Chesterton said, "A dead thing can go with the stream, but only a living thing can go against it."[2] When you are alive in Christ, you feel the tension between following the crowd (and going with the flow) versus living to please God.

Fighting the good fight means you're aware of what you are up against, you'll do the hard work, and only God has power over you. Philippians 2:13 (NLT) says, "For God is working in you, giving you the desire and the power to do what pleases him." Whatever He calls you to do, He'll equip you to do. He'll get you in fighting condition.

Life is full of breathtaking good and heartbreaking evil. Even if you don't feel strong, you can stay in the game. You can make empowering choices. Wherever you are, start there. Don't let a lack of anything keep you from trying, because God takes care of His children.

Seek help, borrow strength, and get yourself physically, mentally, and spiritually healthy. Protect the spirit in your heart and the light in your eyes, because you, my friend, are worth it.

> This is my command—be strong and courageous! Do not be afraid or discouraged. For the LORD your God is with you wherever you go.
>
> JOSHUA 1:9 (NLT)

KNOW YOUR BIGGEST ENEMY

Both times that I've taken a self-defense class, the first topic covered was situational awareness.

Why? Because being unaware of your surroundings makes you an easy target.

Self-defense instructors emphasize trusting your instincts. They tell you to pay attention to red flags and keep your eyes open; if you're walking toward someone who gives you a funny vibe, then change paths and distance yourself, even if it means taking a longer route. They advise you to make eye contact because criminals don't want to be recognized. If you can identify them in a lineup, you lose appeal as a victim.

I discuss this with my daughters so they can recognize evil. *I want them to know they aren't crazy when an event or a person triggers strange feelings or unease.* In Matthew 10:16 (NLT) Jesus said: "Look, I am sending you out as sheep among wolves. So be as shrewd as snakes and harmless as doves." What this means is to be mindful and vigilant. Loving, yet smart. Tender, yet tough—keeping the heart of a child and the mind of an adult.

Sometimes trouble is obvious, and sometimes it hides behind pretty faces and half-truths. At every age we need discernment to see what is and isn't from God. As Charles Spurgeon said, "Discernment is not knowing the difference between right and wrong; it is knowing the difference between right and almost right."[3]

You may think your worst enemy is a human being, but your real enemy, the source of all darkness, is Satan. While he is no match for God, he is a predator. And like all predators, he'll catch his prey off-guard. He likes to attack when you least expect it.

Scripture says:

- Satan is the father of lies. (John 8:44)
- He comes to steal, kill, and destroy. (John 10:10)
- He prowls like a lion, looking for someone to devour. (1 Peter 5:8)
- You can stand against his schemes by putting on the armor of God. (Ephesians 6:11)

- You are not fighting against flesh-and-blood enemies, but against mighty powers and spiritual forces of evil. (Ephesians 6:12)
- Satan will flee if you resist him and obey God. (James 4:7)
- If you belong to God, then you've already won, because God's Spirit in you is greater than Satan's spirit in the world. (1 John 4:4)
- God fights for you against your enemies and gives you victory. (Deuteronomy 20:4)
- The light shines in the darkness, and the darkness can't overcome it. (John 1:5)
- We are more than conquerors through Christ who loved us. (Romans 8:37)
- One day, spiritual warfare will end, and God will create a new heaven and a new earth. (Revelation 21)

The Greek word for devil is *diabolos,* which means "the one who divides." When you feel division in your life, you can assume the diabolos is at work.

He will try to stir the pot, create irreconcilable differences, and fan into flames any anger, irritation, jealousy, or frustration that you feel. Understanding his M.O. helps you not take the bait. While Jesus brings life, the enemy brings death, and whether you sense it or not, we live in a world of spiritual warfare. There are forces trying to separate you (and me) from God.

Thankfully, you don't fight alone. Jesus is always ready to help, and all you have to do is ask. He can strengthen you, empower you, and unite you with allies. He can sharpen your discernment and situational awareness so that your senses and eyes stay open.

Your best weapons in any battle are *armor* and *light.* Put on

God's armor and follow the light, trusting Him as your protector and guide.

> The people who walk in darkness will see a great light. For those who live in a land of deep darkness, a light will shine.
>
> Isaiah 9:2 (NLT)

PREPARE FOR BATTLE

I once heard yelling in my basement that sounded like an ugly fight between two sisters.

As I went to break it up, I discovered it was my nine-year-old daughter screaming at herself. She was mad about her tumbling, and it crushed me to realize how she had started her journey of the battle within.

For years I have loved 2 Corinthians 5:17 (NIV): "Therefore, if anyone is in Christ, the new creation has come: The old has gone, the new is here!" Through Jesus, God makes us new creations. Our old self dies, and we gain new life through Christ. He strengthens us through the Holy Spirit.

There is big hope in this message, yet what often gets excluded from this conversation is the struggle that remains. *Being made new in Christ isn't a one-time deal; God must continuously make us new because we're constantly tempted to resort to our old ways.* Old ways of thinking, acting, and living. Patterns we revert to in moments of weakness. External battles *and* internal battles that weigh us down.

Besides fighting temptations from the enemy, we also fight our old nature. We battle an inner tension as God's spirit calls us in one direction, and our flesh pulls us in another.

Thankfully, Jesus understands. He knows our hearts, fears,

and desires, and He experienced temptation firsthand. In any battle, He is your greatest ally. Here are eight ways to lean into His grace.

1. Put on the armor of God.

Ephesians 6:10–18 is a battle anthem. It praises God as your strength and protector. It empowers you with invisible weapons.

The Message version reads: "God is strong, and he wants you strong. So take everything the Master has set out for you, well-made weapons of the best materials. And put them to use so you will be able to stand up to everything the Devil throws your way. This is no weekend war that we'll walk away from and forget about in a couple of hours. This is for keeps, a life-or-death fight to the finish against the Devil and all his angels.

"Be prepared. You're up against far more than you can handle on your own. Take all the help you can get, every weapon God has issued, so that when it's all over but the shouting you'll still be on your feet. Truth, righteousness, peace, faith, and salvation are more than words. Learn how to apply them. You'll need them throughout your life. God's Word is an *indispensable* weapon. In the same way, prayer is essential in this ongoing warfare. Pray hard and long. Pray for your brothers and sisters. Keep your eyes open. Keep each other's spirits up so that no one falls behind or drops out."

2. Pray.

Prayer leads to spiritual breakthroughs. Your prayers don't return void, and though God doesn't promise quick fixes, He does hear you and respond. A strong prayer life connects you with God and lets you impact the future through prayers that outlive your time on earth.

It is natural to pray for your loved ones, but you can also pray for your adversaries. Ask God to soften their hearts and help you see them through His eyes.

I know a woman who hated her ex-husband's new wife because she tried to turn her own kids against her. Her perspective changed when a church mentor asked if she was praying for this new wife. When she said, "No, why would I do that?" the mentor replied, "If you don't pray for her, who will?" From then on, she prayed for this woman and for healing in their relationship for the sake of her children.

History is full of stories about hearts restored and relationships mended through the power of prayer. Nothing is too far gone for God to redeem.

3. Know why you're fighting.

Fighting just to fight is pointless. Pick your battles wisely, and save your resources for the battles that matter most.

Are you fighting to get yourself in a better place, or to unload rage? Are you seeking truth, or determined to win at any cost? Are you led by the Holy Spirit, or triggered by emotions? Is this fight worth it? Does it detract from another fight with bigger things at stake, like somebody's soul?

4. Know what you're fighting.

As we brainstormed ideas for this book, my editor Stephanie said, "Strength is not being perfect; strength is being self-aware."

Amen. To be strong, you must know yourself and admit your weak points. Doing honest self-reflection helps you identify where the enemy may attack you.

If you envy your friend, for instance, he'll work that angle. If you despise your child's coach, he'll fuel that fire. If you're prone to depression, he'll feed you gloomy thoughts. If you're constantly overwhelmed, he'll find clever ways to make you feel the weight of the world on your shoulders.

While your "hard" may be different than my "hard," we battle common things

- fear
- guilt
- jealousy
- insecurity
- inadequacy
- anxiety
- pessimism
- burnout
- negative thoughts
- poor self-image
- pride
- vanity
- greed
- perfectionism
- people-pleasing

- self-adoration
- self-importance
- materialism
- impatience
- self-loathing
- self-doubt
- shame
- bitterness
- resentment
- apathy
- despair
- a burning need to impress
- a burning need to prove
  our critics wrong

Feeling confident in God's love, despite your ugly truths, is crucial to self-awareness. Ask Him to help you unpack your baggage and love yourself through the process.

5. Bring your secrets to light.

There is an old saying in Alcoholics Anonymous: "You're only as sick as your secrets." In any struggle, it's tempting to withdraw and turn inward, but this puts you at risk for attacks.

You need people praying for you, speaking truth, and guarding you against the enemy. While I don't recommend sharing your secrets randomly, I do believe it's healthy to share them with people you trust.

Dorotheos, a Christian monk and Desert Father, said we have a lot more power to conquer our struggles early (when they are small) and before they become engrained habits. If we depend on our own strength and have nobody to support us, if we don't bring to light everything about ourselves and make a habit of revealing our inner thoughts and seeking godly counsel, then the enemy can make a plaything of us. Just bringing the truth to light makes the devil flee.

He wrote, "We need assistance, we need guidance in addition to God's grace. No one is more wretched, no one is more easily caught unaware, than a man who has no one to guide him along the road to God. Those who have no guidance fall like leaves."[4]

Verbalizing your struggles gets easier with practice. Start with one confidante, and build from there. This will teach your children to be honest too, to not be ashamed of their humanity or wrongly assume that no one would understand them.

If you don't want your kids to struggle alone, let them see you seek help for your struggles.

6. Have an accountability partner.

A respected mom in my community helped each of her four sons form an accountability group in high school with like-minded friends.

Each group met weekly in their basement to admit their recent temptations and missteps. They spoke freely, sharing what they might not feel comfortable saying in front of their parents. These meetings kept them honest and taught them to rely on close friends for accountability and growth.

It's helpful to have someone—your spouse, sister, best friend, therapist, etc.—who holds you accountable and helps you fight your struggles too.

7. Seek wise counsel.

Whenever I feel weak or foggy-minded, God places people around me who are strong and clear-minded. They lend strength and think for me until I can think for myself again.

This is no accident, for God uses and speaks through people. Keep trustworthy and wise people around you. Let them be your moral support and your sounding board, especially if you have toxic thoughts or a relationship that has led you to an unhealthy place.

8. Stay humble.

Pride is the greatest evil, C. S. Lewis said, because it leads to every other vice and is the complete anti-God state of mind.

Sadly, there is no fault that we are more *unconscious* of in ourselves. Lewis wrote, "As long as you are proud you cannot know God. A proud man is always looking down on things and people: and, of course, as long as you are looking down, you cannot see something that is above you."[5]

To receive God's power, you need humility. Scripture reiterates this point:

- Pride comes before a fall. (Proverbs 16:18)
- God opposes the proud and shows favor to the humble. (James 4:6)
- God lifts you up when you humble yourself before Him. (James 4:10)
- God humbles those who exalt themselves, and He exalts those who humble themselves before Him. (Matthew 23:12)

- Pride leads to disgrace; humility brings wisdom. (Proverbs 11:2)
- God gives power to the weak and strength to the powerless. (Isaiah 40:29)
- God's power is made perfect in weakness; you can brag about your weaknesses so the power of Christ works through you. (2 Corinthians 12:9)

Not every "success" comes from God, for Satan is happy to help you succeed at the wrong things. He may even help you build an empire because the higher you rise, the greater your fall will be.

Surprisingly, humility is a weapon to fight the enemy. In the book *Wisdom from Mount Athos,* a monk named Staretz Silouan said that when saints waged war against evil spirits, they conquered them through humility, prayer, and fasting. We should fear pride and vainglory, not evil spirits, because through them we lose grace.

Silouan wrote, "The Lord does not manifest Himself to the proud soul. All the books in the world will not help the proud soul to know the Lord. Her pride will not make way for the grace of the Holy Spirit, and God is known only through the Holy Spirit."[6]

In Scripture, I love the book of Acts because it shows the disciples transform and prepare for battle. After Jesus dies, and before the Holy Spirit comes to live within them, these men are sad, discouraged, and scared. They lock themselves in a room for fear of being killed like their leader.

Then, on Pentecost, Jesus sends the "Advocate" that He promised would arrive after He left (John 16:7). Filled with the Holy Spirit, the disciples become brave and bold. They start the Christian church and embark on an ambitious mission to spread the gospel worldwide and make disciples.

They suffer and get persecuted, and most of them die for their faith, yet they remain undeterred. They know that saving souls is worth this punishment.

This is the marvel of the Holy Spirit. This is what emboldens and equips believers, knowing that even if our bodies get destroyed, our souls live on.

Your battles may catch you off-guard, but not God. He has known every detail since the beginning of time. Let Him help you fight the enemy. Rely on the spiritual armor that no one can diminish or take away.

> What then shall we say to these things? If God is for us, who can be against us?
>
> ROMANS 8:31 (ESV)

SEE THE LIGHT, BE THE LIGHT

My husband has a cousin who spent a week at a well-known monastery in Greece.

He said it was life-changing to live among monks, and as he entered the monastery, an intense warmth surrounded him. He felt enveloped by the Holy Spirit. It created a euphoria unlike any high he had ever known.

This warmth triggered a memory of another experience from years before. What he felt inside the monastery was the exact *opposite* of what he felt while touring an old concentration camp in Germany. Although the camp is now used to teach history, he sensed the evil from its Nazi past. As he walked into that building, the air felt so chilling that his hair stood on end.

Warmth versus chill. Light versus darkness. Morality versus corruption. Sometimes the best way to recognize evil is in comparison to what is good. As you see and sense the contrast, you understand the difference between heaven and hell.

While darkness is real, there is no need to fear it or obsess over it, because God is greater and more worthy of attention. As you worship Him, study His character, and spend time with godly people, your spiritual awareness deepens. Your instincts sharpen, attuning you to what is real.

The better you know God, the harder you are to fool. One analogy that is used to explain this truth is money. Did you know that when bank tellers are trained to recognize counterfeit bills, they study real currency? They become experts on genuine money, and this helps them spot the fakes.

In a similar vein, it's a better use of your time to sit with God, grow your faith, and strengthen your intuition than to give Satan undue attention. Once you recognize the enemy's hand, half the battle is won.

Will you always get it right and choose the best path? Of course not, because you're human, and we all get offtrack. But even when that happens, God can redirect you. He can show a better way. He can comfort you in your troubles so that you can later comfort others.

Accepting this guidance gives purpose to your pain. It deepens your compassion. It makes you a light for those behind you and turns you into a valiant warrior.

In your lifetime, you'll fight many internal and external battles. The outcomes won't depend on you, because you're not in control. God walks with you and before you, giving grace exactly when you need it. Believe in the strength inside you. Remember the victory of eternal life. Pray for the discernment to know which battles are yours to fight.

Two years from now, you'll feel proud of today's efforts to be a brave fighter. You may see your kids become brave fighters too. With every step forward, you inspire those around you. You show them what can be overcome with the heart and resolve of a warrior.

> I have fought the good fight, I have finished the race, I have kept the faith.
>
> 2 TIMOTHY 4:7 (NIV)

What Fighting the Good Fight Models for Your Child

In 2015, my husband died tragically in a plane crash. I became a solo parent to two little girls, ages three and five, and the owner of a commercial construction company in the blink of an eye.

During the heaviest grief imaginable, I had critical choices to make that would define our future. Would I look for the good during the deepest sorrow? Would I allow grief to shape me for the better or succumb to the loneliness and immense pain?

Each morning on the way to school, I prayed with my girls and asked God to show us signs of his goodness—to open our eyes to see, our ears to hear, our hearts to receive. At night, I fell asleep with my hands open, acknowledging that God was in complete control of our lives, and upon waking, I rolled onto my knees and asked Him to carry me through the day, one step at a time, one decision at a time.

I grieved openly before my daughters, allowing us to heal together. I continued John's legacy and learned how to run a construction company to demonstrate resiliency lived out and the ability to conquer fears of inadequacy and failure. I opened my heart again to love to embrace a second story for our family.

Mary Wyatt Crenshaw
mother of two daughters

REFLECTION QUESTIONS

1. What has been your biggest battle? Compare your *before* and *after* self.

2. Has a challenge ever stolen the light from your eyes? What helped you (or is helping you now) bounce back?

3. What do you believe about the enemy? Have you ever felt spiritual warfare or seen signs of an attack? Explain.

4. Who are your safe people? Who listens without judgment? If you don't have safe people yet, who can fill that role?

5. "Two years from now, you'll feel proud of today's efforts to be a brave fighter." What brave steps have you taken lately?

6. Have you ever made a critical choice that defined your future? Explain.

9

EMBRACE YOUR PURPOSE

A Mother Needs to Feel Important

*Ask Jesus what he wants from
you and be brave!*

POPE FRANCIS[1]

M y friend Brooke thought she was taking her child to a routine two-year-old checkup.

But when her daughter's bloodwork looked abnormal, the doctor ordered follow-up tests. From there, a nightmare unfolded as Brooke and her husband learned that their vivacious and spunky child had been diagnosed with childhood cancer.

They were devastated, and while their daughter now thrives as a teenager and has been in remission for years, it was a frightening time of uncertainty. Nobody knew what the future held.

Brooke, a self-proclaimed introvert, shies away from attention. She is most content in her comfort zone of nesting at home. But as thousands of people followed her on CaringBridge.org, where she poured her heart out, Brooke received invitations to share her story in person. She always said *yes* even though she hates public speaking and would get so nervous beforehand that she wouldn't eat for days.

"I'm so grateful for what God has done for us," she told me, "that I want to do something in return for Him."

Her courage intrigued me, and when I told my dad about it, he said, "An introvert can become an extrovert when they do something for God."

Wow. What truth. Little did I know, I'd need this truth myself years later when my first book for teen and tween girls was released and I got invited to speak. As I questioned these opportunities, since public speaking made me nervous, my dad told me, "When you're nervous, you're thinking too much about yourself. Focus instead on your audience. Think about the people you're trying to help and the message you came to share."

His words hit home. And like my friend Brooke, I discovered the secret to being brave is to forget about yourself and focus on helping others. As that happens, you walk into your purpose.

Too often in life we drift aimlessly. Even if we embrace our purpose as moms, we may wrongly believe our purpose is over once our kids leave home. The truth, however, is that your purpose continues until your last breath on earth.

Your purpose is even greater than your calling as a mom.

Pastor Rick Warren wrote a life-changing book on this subject. His opening line, "It's not about you," makes it clear that we exist for God's purposes. *The Purpose-Driven Life* is one of the bestselling books of all time (over 35 million copies sold), and it explains how every human being is uniquely created and gifted to serve their generation. There may be accidental pregnancies, but there are no accidental babies. God does *not* make mistakes.

Warren says:

> You cannot arrive at your life's purpose by starting with a focus on yourself. You must begin with God, your Creator. You exist only because God wills that you exist. You were made *by* God and *for* God—and until you understand that, life will never make sense. It is only in God that we discover our origin, our identity, our meaning, our purpose, our significance, and our destiny. Every other path leads to a dead end.[2]

Throughout your life, God will call you outside your comfort zone. He'll give you assignments outside your wheelhouse and dreams without all the answers. He'll force you to step up and be brave.

Before you dismiss His nudges, ask yourself, "Do I not want

to do this because I'm scared, or because it feels wrong?" If your hesitation is due to fear, pray for help. Seek counsel to discern God's voice, and ask for the grace to do His will.

The reason why we accept God's assignments is in response to His perfect love. Your good work returns to Him what He has already given to you. At every age, you have a purpose, one that fulfills your heart's desire to make a lasting and meaningful difference.

> For we are God's handiwork, created in Christ Jesus to do
> good works, which God prepared in advance for us to do.
>
> EPHESIANS 2:10 (NIV)

TAKE STEPS IN THE RIGHT DIRECTION

When finding your purpose, your direction matters more than your speed.

Many people are going nowhere fast, which is why a few steps in the right direction is better than 10,000 steps in the wrong direction.

Every day, your choices move the needle. You either walk closer to God or you move away. Even small steps of faith add up. They create a trajectory for your life that can launch you in a meaningful direction or toward a dead-end road.

God wants you to live with focus, intention, and vision. Without a vision, people perish, and without focus or intention, you lose sight of your goals and wander.

Fortunately, you don't need a road map or a long-term vision to find purpose. The biggest requirement is a desire to please God. Take one baby step at a time, and your answers will come. You'll find your path and direction.

Here are eight ways to seek purpose and walk in God's will.

1. Do the next right thing.

Emily Freeman has a book and a podcast based on this phrase that's been used by people like Theodore Roosevelt, Mother Teresa, and Reverend Martin Luther King Jr. Adults make over 35,000 decisions daily, and breaking those choices down makes them less overwhelming. Rather than worry about a detailed life plan, focus on doing the next right thing.[3]

2. Trust in small starts.

A marathon runner was asked to name the hardest part of running. He replied, "Putting on my shoes." Sometimes, the main challenge is getting started.

Imagine what is possible and then set small goals. If you long to be an artist, start by painting thirty minutes a day. If you dream of creating a national boys' ministry, lead a local Bible study for your son and his friends. If you'd love to be a real estate agent, invite someone in that field to lunch. If you want to decorate homes, start a notebook with your favorite images from home décor magazines and Pinterest.

Get your feet wet, learn, and grow organically from there.

3. Remember, U-turns are allowed.

If you wake up one day and regret the path that you are on, change direction. Rather than go deeper and waste more time, do a U-turn.

Turn around, look for light, and ask for help from people you admire.

We all get misguided, and we all need people who lead us home. Don't follow up one mistake with another mistake or believe that it's too late. *Christianity is not about perfection;*

it is about transformation and accepting Christ's invitation to change. Even on the cross, Jesus forgave the criminal crucified next to him who repented right before his death. He told the criminal, "I assure you, today you will be with me in paradise" (Luke 23:43, NLT).

God cares more about who you're becoming than who you've been in the past. He meets you in your mess, however ugly it may be. That is the beauty, and miracle, of grace.

4. Disrupt your direction when needed.

A guy I know chose military school for college because he needed discipline. His high school crowd was wild, and since his parents set no rules, he partied with the best of them. Deep down, however, he knew that he'd never achieve his life goals staying on this track.

Choosing a military school was an act of self-love that helped him ultimately build a happy and healthy marriage, family, and career. His decision paid off, and had he not made it, he feels certain that he would have fallen into addiction like his two best friends from childhood.

You may be a product of your past, but you're not chained to your past. Stay open to new insights and directions that help you thrive.

5. Make choices that give you peace.

A clear conscience is the softest pillow, and you often know what step to take by how it makes you feel deep down.

Maybe you're tempted to leave your job for a new job with a better salary, yet something about the new company doesn't sit well with you. Maybe you want to say *no* to chairing the school fundraiser, yet you can't shake the feeling that God has called you to it. Tune into your feelings of both unease and peace. Make choices that help you sleep well at night and feel good about your path.

6. Be patient.

Most of us wish that God would deliver all of the answers up front. We want to know The Plan, yet we only get parts of the puzzle.

You never know at the start of a journey what that journey will entail. Only as the puzzle comes together does it slowly make sense. Your biggest breakthroughs will come not when you're coasting along, but when you're struggling. When you feel lost, frustrated, or tempted to quit, you become open to guidance and desperate for divine intervention.

This builds humility. It makes you depend on God as more than a Google map. Your purpose won't develop magically overnight, but with patience, it will become more clear.

7. Choose good mentors.

It's been said that when you choose your advisor, you choose your advice. Ask five people for advice, and you'll get five different answers. You may get opposite answers.

For this reason, I believe in choosing mentors who 1) know you and your history and 2) know God and His character. Armed with this, they can offer relevant counsel while also understanding what may be stirring in your heart.

Your character matters more than your goals, so choose mentors and influences who contribute to the vision of who you hope to be.

8. Notice a need and respond.

In a podcast titled "Many Have Contemplated Suicide," a monk named Father Abbot Tryphon says that according to a recent study from the Centers for Disease Control, one in four young adults ages eighteen to twenty-four had contemplated suicide in the previous thirty days.

Father Tryphon says we all can contribute to the health of others. Walking through life with a smile on our face and a song in our heart may help others stay afloat in one of the most difficult periods of history. By keeping our mind and heart in a good place, we can be a lifeline.

He shares a story about a young man he met while hiking up a remote trail. The young man was sitting on a log, deep in thought, and Father Tryphon apologized for startling him. He could tell something was wrong, so he commented on the beauty of God's creation.

The young man asked Father Tryphon if he was an angel. The monk sat down beside him and offered half his lunch. A few moments later, the young man turned to Father Tryphon and showed him a revolver. He'd come to this remote location to kill himself, and when he saw a monk with a long white beard and a black robe, he thought God had sent an angel. He confessed that he'd been praying for God to forgive him for what he was about to do.

Father Tryphon assured him that he was no angel, but he *was* sent by God as a messenger. *He told this young man that he was loved, God had a plan for his life, and this period of despair would soon pass.* The young man handed Father Tryphon his revolver, and the monk emptied the bullets and put them in his backpack. They had a long conversation and walked back to their cars together. The young man promised to return the revolver to his dad and tell him about his plan that got thwarted after an encounter with a monk.

Father Tryphon often thinks about that young man and wonders what may have happened if he hadn't smiled and shared his sandwich. To this day, he feels blessed that God allowed him to be His messenger on a lonely trail.[4]

All around you, every day, people are struggling. God is simply asking you to notice a need and respond. Be a messenger and make time for special encounters. You never know when you may alter someone's life and discover a new purpose on a remote path.

In Christianity, we are defined by our future, not by our past. God doesn't give vision without provision or purpose without power. As you consider life's big questions—*Why am I here? What is my purpose? How can I make my life count?*—remember how God has it all figured out. Keep praying for answers. Pay attention to nudges. Stay faithful in the little assignments, and be ready for the big assignments that may later come your way.

> His master replied, "Well done, good and faithful servant! You have been faithful with a few things; I will put you in charge of many things. Come and share your master's happiness!"
>
> MATTHEW 25:23 (NIV)

RUN YOUR RACE

One cohort that I have grown to love is young adults in their early twenties with visions and dreams for their future.

The ones I meet have a passion to help the boys and girls behind them. What impresses me most is their energy, passion, and teachability. They know what they want, they're sure of their ideas, and they're fired up to make things happen.

These young adults remind me that having vision allows

people to help you. You know who to talk to and what questions to ask. You meet people who will root for you, guide you, and catch your contagious energy.

Chances are, you once had visions and dreams. You had bright-eyed wonder and suspense about your future. But motherhood rearranged your priorities. You discovered the pinnacle of purpose in raising your children, and what on earth could compare to that?

I can't speak for all moms, but I realized early on how nothing will ever bring me the same joy, fulfillment, or sense of purpose as being a mother. My kids and my husband are the best chapters of my life, and if I died tomorrow, I wouldn't have a single regret about embracing them as my primary purpose.

At the same time, I may live another forty or fifty years. I'm launching teenagers and wondering what my life will look like in its second act. My family will always be my greatest purpose, but once my nest is empty, I'll have more time and energy. I'll have more head space and heart space to serve God.

The question is: What next? How do we parlay our experiences as women and mothers into fresh callings and pursuits? Clearly, I have my writing, yet even with that, I feel somewhat lost. I struggle to imagine possibilities after being out of practice so long.

The dreaming that once came naturally to me no longer does. Sometimes I wonder if my ship has sailed.

Many women feel this way. I know so many smart mothers who underestimate themselves and believe they no longer have talents. They feel like they have no purpose after their kids leave home. I get it because I've felt it.

When you've been out of college or the workplace for twenty to thirty years; when you've lost your edge because you've been stretched, pulled, and loved into realness like the Velveteen

Rabbit; when your brain is so tired and fried that you can't remember what you ate for lunch and you worry that you have dementia—well, it's easy to assume you have nothing to offer.

But here is your hidden advantage: your mother's heart. You may not have the speed, sharp-mindedness, or charisma of youth, but you do have an amazing heart. You have an outlook that no one can teach through school or a seminar. You've cultivated your mother's heart through blood, sweat, and tears, and it lets you give our world *exactly* what it needs now.

Your other hidden advantage is the Holy Spirit. Through it, God works miracles. None of us are here to make ourselves famous; we're here to make Jesus famous. And when your visions are inspired by that, and your drive is inspired by the Holy Spirit, your purpose will surface.

In Scripture, God says to run your race with endurance, fix your eyes on Jesus, and remember the hostility He faced so you don't grow weary or lose heart (Hebrews 12:1–3). He shows many examples of using ordinary people for extraordinary purposes—people like Peter, who constantly messed up and even denied knowing Jesus, yet was chosen to lead the first church.

Even with His disciples, Jesus didn't pick the smartest, most talented men. He wasn't looking for superstars. Instead, he looked for humble, teachable hearts. Your heart matters more than your ability, and if you cooperate with God's grace, He'll give you the Holy Spirit and use you for good.

How does this look in real life? How do you run your race or cast a vision when you feel unequipped or when you're barely hanging on?

Here is how: You envision who you hope to be. You consider the example you hope to set. You picture yourself standing tall and pulling up others from the pit of despair. You remember this from Christine Caine: "God uses rescued people to rescue people."[5]

Even when you struggle, you have a purpose. You never know who may be watching or taking notes on the way that you handle your trials.

We all need visions of who we can be. Visions help us set a high bar and rise to our potential. Look to Jesus as the ultimate inspiration (studying His life, His thinking, and His sacrifices), and ask how you can be brave for Him.

Running your race means living the life that *you* were born to live. We all get distracted, and even when you're on the right track, there may be impediments that trip you up. Here are a few

- *Comparison:* just glancing at the woman next to you who is running faster and better can trigger your insecurity.
- *Envy:* the moral support you need is often undermined by competition and forgetting that you and other women are on the same team.
- *Perfectionism:* nothing crushes your spirit like impossible expectations.
- *People-pleasing:* nothing gets you off track more than chasing human applause.
- *Boredom and disillusionment:* when your race feels monotonous, you may miss the fire and novelty of starting anew.
- *Overconfidence:* as you catch your stride, it's easy to lose humility.
- *Lack of confidence:* as you stumble or fall, it can mess with your mind.
- *Fear:* whether it's fear of failure, rejection, judgment, or looking dumb, it can paralyze you.

I have a friend who loves to write, but she put writing on the back burner to work a pharmaceutical sales job and provide for her family.

After running into a male friend from college, who knew her as the girl with a passion for words, not the mom with a sensible job, she realized how much she missed writing when he brought up the writing dreams she once talked about with stars in her eyes.

She'd forgotten those plans, and she missed that girl who dreamed. After this encounter, she began to write again. She used her waiting time in doctor's offices to work on a manuscript.

Where there is a will, there is a way. And when your purpose isn't clear, look at your passions. What brings you to life? What makes you lose track of time? What feeds your soul? What is your place of peace? What old dreams have slipped through the cracks? What would you do if you weren't afraid?

Now may not be the time to rekindle an old passion. But even if you're waiting, you can think about what once stole your heart and remember the girl with visions and dreams. At every age, she is relevant to your story. She is a clue to the direction your life is meant to take.

> Keep your eyes on *Jesus*, who both began and finished this race we're in. Study how he did it. Because he never lost sight of where he was headed—that exhilarating finish in and with God—he could put up with anything along the way: Cross, shame, whatever. And now he's *there*, in the place of honor, right alongside God. When you find yourselves flagging in your faith, go over that story again, item by item, that long litany of hostility he plowed through. *That* will shoot adrenaline into your souls!
>
> HEBREWS 12:2–3 (MSG)

KEEP YOUR OPTIONS OPEN

Throughout your life, your purpose will evolve. It may look different from one season or one day to the next.

Embrace today's assignments while knowing that tomorrow's assignments may require new skills. God may plant new desires and convictions in your heart. He may ask you to steward a new calling, at least temporarily.

Staying open and obedient will give you a purpose even through transitions. Whatever God asks of you, it points to the same goal: to draw hearts to Him.

God has equipped you with unique talents, insights, experiences, and stories. While your life is God's gift to you, what you do with your life is your gift back to Him. So often, we *tell* God what we want rather than *ask* what He wants of us. We let assignments pass us by because we're scared, preoccupied, or lazy—or because we feel unqualified.

But since every assignment prepares you for the next assignment, ignoring one can set you back. It can keep you from living your best life possible.

Thankfully, God is gracious. He presents new mercies each morning and new chances to be brave. He allows us to serve by giving our time, talent, and treasure. He turns introverts into extroverts by drawing us out of our shell.

Again, the same spirit that raised Jesus from the dead is what empowers Christ believers. It births new goals, new visions, and new dreams. In every assignment, God provides, and He teaches lessons that won't hit home when life feels easy or predictable.

Outside your comfort zone is where you learn to trust, dig deep, and lean into your faith. It is where you discover a new side of yourself and branch out in a new direction.

"I am the vine; you are the branches. If you remain in me and I in you, you will bear much fruit; apart from me you can do nothing."

JOHN 15:5 (NIV)

What Embracing Your Purpose Models for Your Child

After having four children in seven years, I thought my career as a magazine editor, content creator, and stylist was over since, it involved travel and days away from home.

While my husband was wonderful and very engaged, raising four children required all hands on deck. I wanted to be fully present in the season of babies and toddlers, and I embraced my new job within the confines of our home.

But as my kids grew up and started real school, I longed to find a purpose beyond motherhood. I missed being creative, and I knew that reigniting my creative side would make me a better me—*and* a better mom.

After many wide-awake nights in bed and some brainstorming with a friend who is now my business partner, The Southern Coterie was born. Founded in 2011, it has taken off and surpassed our wildest dreams. What we've seen it do in the lives of our community has been extraordinary.

Through an annual convention in Sea Island, Georgia, female entrepreneurs and creatives from across the country have formed authentic friendships and productive business connections. They mentor, empower, and cheer each other on, cultivating a vibrant community of females whose passion projects change the world.

For over fifteen years, I've kept a tattered "Parent's Prayer Card" in a box on my nightstand. One prayer asks that "our children use Godly wisdom and discernment in selecting their friends, for friends and peers do make a difference." I've always seen this truth manifest in my children's lives, and now, I witness it in my work life.

Whenever I see the smart, kind, and talented ladies of the Southern C positively impact each other's lives, I feel like a proud mom. And what I hope to model for my children is the importance of choosing a passion project that benefits, serves, and helps others. I hope my daughter sees the spectacular power of women lifting up women, and I hope my sons see how capable, brilliant, and remarkable women can be.

Whitney Wise Long
mom of three sons and one daughter

REFLECTION QUESTIONS

1. Name a time when God called you outside your comfort zone. Did you obey or ignore His nudge?

2. Do you believe your direction matters more than your speed? Why or why not?

3. What fears keep you from living out your purpose?

4. "Take one baby step at a time, and your answers will come. You'll find your path and direction." Have your small steps ever opened a big door? Have you ever waited so long you gave up? Explain.

5. Do you believe hard times serve a purpose? Has God ever comforted you in your troubles so you can comfort others?

6. Think about your purpose beyond motherhood. What talents or strengths can you share outside your home?

10

LIVE IN HOPE

A Mother Needs to Feel Optimistic

*Although the world is full of suffering,
it is also full of the overcoming of it.*

HELEN KELLER[1]

The day before my twenty-ninth birthday began with utter bliss—and ended with gut-wrenching pain.

Just three days before, I'd learned that I was pregnant, and Harry and I were ecstatic.

We laughed and dreamed as we drove to the beach to spend a weekend with his friends. Already we felt like proud parents. We couldn't stop talking about baby names, the nursery, and starting our own family.

Then, as we stopped to see a friend, our excitement came to a halt. As I used my friend's restroom, I saw the startling red signs of a miscarriage.

I called my doctor, and he said if it was a miscarriage, there was nothing I could do to stop it. Instead of driving home, he advised us to go to the beach, take it easy, enjoy the weekend as best we could, and see him on Monday.

Harry and I held out hope, but when the bleeding continued for hours, we knew it wasn't good. Around midnight the cramps kicked in, and as Harry ran to the store to buy me ibuprofen, I curled up in bed and cried like a baby over this treasure we lost on my twenty-ninth birthday. It was one of the most disappointing and jolting days of my life.

It had taken us a year to conceive, so we kept an appointment that I'd scheduled before we got pregnant to see a doctor who could run some tests. He uncovered a cause for concern, and he grimly predicted that getting pregnant again might be difficult.

My lifelong dream was to be a mom, and to suddenly question that possibility triggered deep sadness and fear. What if our pregnancy was a fluke? What if it never happened again? How would we afford adoption when money was already tight after paying graduate school tuition?

It was a lonely season of waiting, praying, and doubting. I learned a lot about myself and trusting God's plan as I attended baby showers for friends and often felt like an outsider when the conversation turned to kids. By God's grace I got pregnant six months later with my oldest daughter, Ella. Around her first birthday I got pregnant again, only to miscarry this baby before Christmas.

Once again, my heart was heavy, and though it made a huge difference having Ella to hold, I also felt the grief of her losing a brother or sister.

Looking back now, it is clear God had a plan. Over the course of my thirties, I birthed four beautiful baby girls, and even if we had not conceived them, I know my prayers to be a mom would have been answered. At the time, however, I couldn't see past the unknowns. I only saw one road, the most common road to motherhood, and if it didn't work out, the future looked dismal and dark.

My faith was not as deep then as it is now, yet it took trials like this to deepen it. What I wish I could tell my younger self is that God takes care of His people. His plan is good, perfect, and always on time. His vision is bolder and grander than any tunnel vision we get, and if we wait patiently, He'll author a better story than any story we could write.

I'd also tell my younger self that life is full of mysteries, and we'll never get full answers to suffering on this side of heaven. But what we do know, as believers, is the best is yet to come. Faith means being sure of what we hope for and certain of what we do not see (Hebrews 11:1).

Still, hope can feel nonexistent during times of loss. Our culture of doom and gloom only compounds the problem. We are surrounded by negativity in media and pop culture, and many popular movies, books, and works of art leave us feeling terribly depressed because they use the framework of our visible world to process sad events. They show no light at the end of the tunnel, no purpose behind the pain, no hope for the future.

If we believe this world is all there is, that how we feel today is how we'll always feel, that we'll never be happy unless our prayers get answered *exactly* the way we hope, that there is no afterlife to anticipate, that suffering is as senseless as it appears, then we'll despair. We'll stay stuck in hopeless places.

But through Jesus, God births *hope*. He shines a light that conquers darkness and death. A Christian's hope boils down to three key words: *He is risen*. Seeing the world through this framework changes everything.

Without Jesus, hope depends on our circumstances. With Jesus, hope eclipses our circumstances.

Life on earth feels permanent, yet it is fleeting. Our real home is in heaven, and the ache in your heart that never goes away, that earthly joys and blessings can only temporarily quench, is really a longing for heaven. God created you to crave Him, and He placed eternity in your heart as a homing device to draw you home toward Him.

Feeling dissatisfied with this world reminds us that we were made for more. We are walking toward our final destination, where perfect peace, love, and joy exist.

C. S. Lewis said, "If I find in myself a desire which no experience in this world can satisfy, the most probable explanation is that I was made for another world."[2] Remembering this fuels hope. *It assures us that no trial lasts forever, and any joy we do experience only foreshadows what is still ahead.*

We always have reason to hope, and these promises back up this truth:

- Anyone who believes in Jesus will have eternal life. (John 3:16)
- Hope is an anchor for the soul. (Hebrews 6:19)
- Hope does not disappoint. (Romans 5:5)
- Hope comes from God, and the soul finds rest in Him alone. (Psalm 62:5)
- Today's sufferings can't compare to the glory that is coming. (Romans 8:18)
- No eye has seen, no ear has heard, and no mind has imagined what God has prepared for those who love him. (1 Corinthians 2:8–9)
- Three things last forever: faith, hope, and love. The greatest is love. (1 Corinthians 13:13)
- If we do good and don't give up, we'll reap blessings at the right time. (Galatians 6:9)
- When we grieve, we shouldn't grieve like those who have no hope, for we believe in Jesus. (1 Thessalonians 4:13–14)
- Those who hope in the LORD will renew their strength. They will soar like eagles, run and not grow weary, walk and not be faint. (Isaiah 40:30–31)
- Faithful servants will share in God's joy. (Matthew 25:21)
- God blesses those who patiently endure testing and temptation. Afterward, they'll receive the crown of life that God has promised to those who love Him. (James 1:12)
- Even if we don't understand what Jesus is doing now, we will one day. (John 13:7)
- After we have suffered a while, God will restore us and make us strong, firm, and steadfast. (1 Peter 5:10)
- The things we see will soon be gone, but the things we can't see will last forever. When the earthly tent we live in is destroyed, we will have an eternal house in heaven made by God. (2 Corinthians 4:18–5:1)

- Everyone born of God overcomes the world. (1 John 5:4)
- One day, God will make everything new. He will create a new order with no tears, no sorrow, no suffering. (Revelation 21:3–6)

God brings new life from heartache, and just as the grief of Good Friday preceded the joy of Easter Sunday, today's trials may lead to miracles. It is only Friday, and Sunday is coming. The darkness in between can feel like light years, and you may need years (or decades) to feel hope again, but that hope is worth fighting for. It is worth remembering how the *first thing* God did after creating the heavens and the earth was bring light into the darkness.

He began the story of humanity by setting the stage for the light of Jesus.

Darkness may be part of your story, but it isn't the end of your story. Circumstances come and go, but God is forever. Put your trust in Him, not what happens to you. Fix your eyes on what is real, and when you feel scared of the unknowns, cling to the virtue of hope.

> "For I know the plans I have for you," says the LORD. "They are plans for good and not for disaster, to give you a future and a hope."
>
> JEREMIAH 29:11 (NLT)

DARE TO HOPE

One of my favorite children's books is Max Lucado's *The Oak Inside the Acorn*.[3]

The book is about an acorn that becomes a big, strong oak tree. Early on, the acorn feels like a failure. He tries to grow oranges like the orange trees and flowers like the rose bush, but with no success. He wonders what must be wrong with him to be so different from the plants he sees.

As the acorn evolves into a small tree that grows branches, his potential manifests. Slowly the acorn realizes and embraces his God-given purpose.

Lucado's message is clear: Just as the destiny of an oak tree is contained in a tiny acorn, there is a miracle inside of you. It takes patience, time, and obedience for this miracle to unfold. You will struggle as you wait and wonder why you're not like anyone else.

As your story plays out and your experiences shape you, your purpose gains clarity. You start to view your uniqueness in relation to your calling.

Philippians 1:6 (NLT) says, "And I am certain that God, who began the good work within you, will continue his work until it is finally finished on the day when Christ Jesus returns." Every human being is a lifelong work in progress. Until your last breath on earth, God will try to make you (and me) more like Jesus. No event is a waste because it all can be used to cultivate Christlike character.

Living in hope makes pain bearable. It reminds you to not discount the season you are in.

Even if you only see black, you could be on the brink of a miracle. You might be like the acorn buried in soil. If that soil is life-giving, hope abounds. Just dig deep and do your part, and then wait for the breakthrough moment where you rise and see the light.

Many people believe they are victims of life. They feel helpless against their circumstances. But hope's crucial component is agency, believing the future will be better than the present, and you have some power to make it so.[4] It is important to know you can influence the future through your choices, prayers, faith, and perspective. Whatever circumstances you face, you get to choose your outlook and attitude.

The quickest way to find hope is to look at Jesus. The quickest way to lose hope is to look at your circumstances. In the Bible, Peter walks on water when his eyes stay on Jesus. But when his attention shifts to the wind that is blowing against him, he gets frightened and begins to sink. He gets reprimanded for his lack of faith (Matthew 14:22–32).

All of us are like Peter, aren't we? Instead of marveling over the miracle—the fact that we can suddenly do the impossible!—we get distracted by the wind. We feel fear and doubt and start to sink. We let our minds wander and get distracted. We fail to notice the grace in our lives.

Thankfully, God is patient. He helps us up again and again and again. Step forward with courage and live in hope. Notice the light you're walking toward, and when you feel like your story is over, remember the miracle inside of you.

> Then Christ will make his home in your hearts as you trust in him. Your roots will grow down into God's love and keep you strong.
>
> EPHESIANS 3:17 (NLT)

SEE YOU IN PARADISE

The light of Jesus is stronger than darkness, even the darkness of death.

Still, finding hope in heartache may take time. When you and I were young, hope came naturally. We had our entire lives before us, open roads of opportunity, and the prospect of what might happen felt like the joy of Christmas morning.

But now, with so much life and mileage behind us, plus the baggage we've picked up, we can wonder if our best days are over.

We can feel regret and disappointment over dashed expectations, missed opportunities, and unrealized dreams. We can look in the rearview mirror and long to go back. We can feel so overwhelmed by events that hope stays in the past.

Add to this a culture where misery loves company, and where you may be ridiculed or misunderstood for being hopeful, and it becomes clear why you need stubborn hope to survive dark times.

God promised eternal life before the world began, and God doesn't lie (Titus 1:2). Every morning when the sun rises, as the light of a new day overcomes the darkness of the night before, His faithfulness shows. Never in history has the sun *not* risen. If you wait patiently, you will see light. Whether your first glimmer comes from a sunrise, a conversation, an open door, a revelation, an answered prayer, or a phone call, it all points to the same thing.

Hope.

Living in hope takes courage. It requires you to keep putting one foot forward and aim to finish strong. ***Regardless of what happens today, tomorrow is a new day.*** It's another chance to get it right and glorify God. Let this prospect fill you with hope and curiosity. Run toward Jesus and keep your eyes on the prize that awaits you on the other side.

Therefore, since we have such a hope, we are very bold.

2 CORINTHIANS 3:12 (NIV)

What Living in Hope Models for Your Child

My beloved friend was six months pregnant with her third child when she was diagnosed with breast cancer. The news stunned her community.

Incredibly brave, and sacrificing her health for her baby girl's health, she waited to be treated until after the delivery. In her final months of pregnancy, family and friends united in prayer, asking God to heal her. Many days we felt hopeless. I felt God continually challenging me to release her and put my hope in Him.

The baby arrived safely, and she was named Hope. Soon after, my friend began treatment. We prayed fervently, yet it quickly became clear that the cancer had progressed and spread. We could only pray, wait, and ask God for a miracle.

A month later, she left this earth to be with Jesus. I had never felt such relentless grief. Besides mourning this friend who I adored, I felt deep pain and heartache for her family.

One verse I have always loved is Romans 8:28 (NIV): "And we know that in all things God works for the good of those who love him, who have been called according to his purpose." Through my friend's sickness and passing, God deepened my understanding of this verse. I've often seen God redeem a trial or tragedy, but with my friend's death, I haven't seen redemption clearly. The only "good" I see is the promise of eternal life. The only hope I have is Jesus.

Because of what He did on the cross, we'll see my friend again. We'll spend eternity together. We have a hope that conquers death!

My family spent four summers with this friend, and my daughters loved her. They witnessed her brave trust in the Lord and her confidence in eternal life. Even at the end, my friend had hope, and even as I grieved, I had hope too. My prayer is that my girls remember this and build their lives on the hope of heaven and the redemption still to come.

Leann Hannan Hanes
mother of three girls

REFLECTION QUESTIONS

1. What heartache from your past made you doubt or lose hope? What would you tell your younger self?

2. Have you ever felt stubborn hope? Explain.

3. Who in your life exudes hope? How has it rubbed off?

4. Have you ever felt peace by looking at Jesus rather than your circumstances? Tell your story.

5. "Hope's crucial component is agency." Do you believe you have agency in your life, or do you feel powerless against your circumstances?

6. Have you ever faced a situation where Jesus was your only hope? If so, how did it change your faith and attitude toward heaven?

CONCLUSION

In my rookie days as a mom, I ignored the advice on self-care.

Quite honestly, I thought it sounded self-indulgent—like an excuse to take bubble baths and visit the spa—and I didn't feel like I needed it. I assumed my early exuberance would always exist. I started my journey as a Giver ready to crush my parenting goals. Little did I know, there would be days that crushed *me*.

Fast-forward twenty years, and I know better. I am older and wiser, and I feel the wear and tear of engaging in a lifelong marathon. Only now do I get the analogy about mothers putting on their oxygen mask first to take care of their family. How can we help anyone if we get knocked out? *What good are we to those we love if we end up on a stretcher?*

If you've parented long enough, then you've learned firsthand why your wellness matters. You've felt the pain (or consequences) of devaluing your wellness. Whether your wake-up call came from a diagnosis, an illness, a breakdown, an issue with your child or spouse, depression, anxiety, or simply feeling depleted and numb, it most likely unveiled this truth:

Mothers are humans too. We require love, compassion, rest, and renewal. Taking care of our needs strengthens us as Givers. It equips us for the road ahead and breeds a second wind that allows us to better love, protect, and serve our family.

Your role as a mother is monumentally important, but you are more than just a mom. You are more than a wife, daughter, sister, CEO, or friend. Above all, you are a child of God. You have inherent worth and dignity. You have infinite value as a human being.

It is easy to lose yourself and your footing in the journey of motherhood. It is tempting to postpone your care and wellness until you have more time and energy. But demands on your time will always exist, so rather than shelve your health and pay the price later, make a habit of checking in using this book as your guide.

The ten chapters of *More Than a Mom* offer a framework to stay on a healthy path. They encourage action toward creating a balanced life. They inspire self-reflection and hope. They give you permission to better yourself and develop as a whole person. My prayer is that you'll incorporate these habits in the months and years ahead:

1. Know Your Worth
2. Rest
3. Build Uplifting Friendships
4. Conquer Stress and Anxiety with Truth
5. Choose Joy
6. Quit the Negative Self-Talk
7. Make Peace with Your Body
8. Fight the Good Fight
9. Embrace Your Purpose
10. Live in Hope

As you blaze your path toward wellness, you set a positive example. You give your children a blueprint for their journey as Givers. One day, they'll be the parents and adults pushing past limits and dismissing warnings about self-care. They may assume they are fine until they reach the end of themselves, when an injury, crisis, heartache, or breaking point brings them to their knees.

In these moments, they'll understand why their health matters. *They'll recall the steps you took to stay healthy for your family.* They'll remember how you weren't ashamed to admit what needed attention. Most importantly, they may invite Jesus into their journey because of what you modeled.

As a mom, you want the best for your loved ones. You hope to be *your* best for your loved ones. Life is too short to settle for unhealthy patterns and positions, and as you work on your wellness, you gain the ability to tell your children, "Do as I am doing" rather than "Do as I say."

Motherhood requires a parallel journey to also take care of yourself. Some of your hardest days as a parent are also your hardest days as a human, so go easy on yourself when you can. Lower your expectations and practice grace and self-compassion. Listen to your body, tend to your needs, and know that you can still move forward at a slower, more gracious pace.

God is with you, God is in you, and God is for you. He can help you become the mother and Giver you hope to be—and the human you deserve to be.

A final word: Be strong in the Lord and in his mighty power.

Ephesians 6:10 (nlt)

NOTES

Introduction

1. Christine Caine quotation, Facebook, December 28, 2020, https://bit.ly/3r3X32w.
2. Dr. Daniel J. Siegel and Dr. Tina Payne Bryson, *The Power of Showing Up: How Parental Presence Shapes Who Our Kids Become and How Their Brains Get Wired*, tinabryson.com, https://bit.ly/2YK5bsN.
3. Dr. Tina Payne Bryson quotation, Twitter, August 10, 2020, https://bit.ly/3u2ZiFB.

Chapter 1: Know Your Worth

1. Dr. Tim Keller quotation, Facebook, February 8, 2017, https://bit.ly/35OdUhj.
2. A. W. Tozer quotation, Twitter, June 8, 2015, https://bit.ly/35KQVUs.
3. Dr. Henry Cloud and Dr. John Townsend, *Boundaries* (Grand Rapids: Zondervan, 1992), 39.
4. Dr. Brené Brown, "Listening to Shame," TED Ideas Worth Spreading, March 2012, https://bit.ly/3ar9kIV.

Chapter 2: Rest

1. Aundi Kolber, *Try Softer* (Carol Stream, IL: Tyndale House Publishers, 2020), 115.

2. Kendra Cherry, "How Multitasking Affects Productivity and Brain Health," Verywell Mind, March 26, 2020, https://bit.ly/2LUltvY.

3. Jenna Fletcher, "Why Sleep Is Essential for Health," Medical News Today, March 31, 2019, https://bit.ly/3pnjw9o.

4. Arianna Huffington, "6 Rules for Better Sleep, According to Arianna Huffington," Time.com, April 19, 2016, https://bit.ly/35OyUot.

5. Liz Mineo, "Good Genes Are Nice, but Joy Is Better," *The Harvard Gazette*, April 11, 2017, https://bit.ly/2M3bogs.

Chapter 3: Build Uplifting Friendships

1. Dr. Vivek H. Murthy, *Together* (New York: HarperCollins Publishers, 2020), 53.

2. Murthy, 8, xvi, 11.

3. Mark Shea, "The Opposite of Love . . . " *National Catholic Register*, June 22, 2011, https://www.ncregister.com/blog/the-opposite-of-love.

4. "Blue Zones: 15 Things We Can Learn from People Who Live to 100," Happy Mammoth, February 1, 2019, https://bit.ly/3jPo2wh.

5. Kari Kampakis, *Love Her Well* (Nashville: W Publishing, 2020), 28.

6. Dr. Tim Keller quotation, Twitter, October 5, 2019, https://bit.ly/3bMyiDj.

7. Liz Mineo, "Good Genes Are Nice, But Joy Is Better," *The Harvard Gazette*, April 11, 2017, https://bit.ly/3qpImq7; and Zameena Mejia, "Harvard's Longest Study of Adult Life Reveals How You Can Be Happier and More Successful," CNBC.com, March 20, 2018, https://cnb.cx/2OJSI6N.

Chapter 4: Conquer Stress and Anxiety with Truth

1. Sissy Goff quotation, Instagram, November 4, 2020, https://bit.ly/2LvfQEN.

2. "Stress vs. Anxiety: How to Tell the Difference," Medical News Today, April 24, 2020, https://bit.ly/3x9hRt1.
3. Anxiety & Depression Association of America, https://bit.ly/2NuyVaM.
4. Emilia Benton, "What Is the 4–7–8 Breathing Technique and How Do You Do It?" *Women's Health Online*, May 18, 2020, https://bit.ly/2NdZBfJ.
5. Dr. Nancy Moyer, "Amygdala Hijack: When Emotion Takes Over," Healthline, April 22, 2019, https://bit.ly/2XKyYkD.
6. Sarah Young, *Jesus Calling Daily Devotional,* October 17, 2020, https://bit.ly/2XMl1T5.
7. Dr. Robert Epstein, "What Makes a Good Parent?" *Scientific American Mind,* November/December 2010, https://bit.ly/38Su8rY.
8. Diane Allen, *Pray, Hope, and Don't Worry: True Stories of Padre Pio Book 1,* Padre Pio Press, 2013, https://amzn.to/3qym71n.

Chapter 5: Choose Joy

1. Henri Nouwen quotation, "Joy," Henrinouwen.org, https://bit.ly/3ipcy1U.
2. Zoya Gervis, "The Average American Spends 24 Days a Year Dreaming About a Vacation," *New York Post,* October 24, 2019, https://bit.ly/3nS1HhZ.
3. Dr. Lisa Damour, "Dear Teenagers, Here's How to Protect Your Emotional Well-Being," *The New York Times,* September 29, 2020, https://nyti.ms/38O7wbY.
4. Dr. Lisa Damour, *Under Pressure* (New York: Ballantine Books, 2019), XVI.
5. Michael Rocque, "Megan Rapinoe Did Not Stomp on the Flag. Here's Why People Got Outraged Regardless," Newsweek.com, July 12, 2019, https://bit.ly/2LYamSG.
6. Sheila Walsh, *It's Okay to Not Be Okay* (Grand Rapids: Baker Books, 2018), 183.

7. Hannah Brockhaus, "Joy Is More than Emotion, It Is a Gift of the Holy Spirit, Pope Francis Says," Catholic News Agency, April 16, 2020, https://bit.ly/2M39GM4.

Chapter 6: Quit the Negative Self-Talk

1. Jennie Allen, *Get Out of Your Head* (Colorado Springs: Waterbrook, 2020), 4.
2. Marie Kondo, *The Life-Changing Magic of Tidying Up: The Japanese Art of Decluttering and Organizing* (New York: Ten Speed Press, 2014), https://amzn.to/2XKaO9O.
3. Joshua Becker, "21 Surprising Statistics That Reveal How Much Stuff We Actually Own," *Becoming Minimalist*, https://bit.ly/3suD5PP.
4. Restore Ministries, Head to Heart Podcast with Julie Sparkman, https://apple.co/3qlJGtY.
5. Courtney E. Ackerman, MA, "What Is Neuroplasticity? A Psychologist Explains," Positive Psychology, December 10, 2020, https://bit.ly/3nOvGat.
6. Kirsten Nunez, "Fight, Flight, Freeze: What This Response Means," Healthline, February 21, 2020, https://www.healthline.com/health/mental-health/fight-flight-freeze.
7. Meditate definition, Google dictionary, https://bit.ly/37KXF6b.
8. Sam Storms, "10 Ways to Effectively Practice Biblical Meditation," Crosswalk.com, March 19, 2018, https://bit.ly/3ilsYYU.
9. Catechism of the Catholic Church, Part Four, Christian Prayer, http://www.scborromeo.org/ccc/p4s1.htm.
10. Dr. Michele Borba, *Thrivers: The Surprising Reasons Why Some Kids Struggle and Others Shine* (New York: G. P. Putnam, 2021), 248.

Chapter 7: Make Peace with Your Body

1. Karen Asp, "50 Body Positivity Quotes, Because It Isn't Easy to Love Your Body 24/7," Parade.com, November 2020, https://bit.ly/3quNrgU.

2. Brittany Tarwater, "Eating Disorders on the Rise During COVID-19 Pandemic, Experts Say," WYMT.com, Nov. 9, 2020, https://bit.ly/35LMqt0.

3. Jenna Birch, "Could Social Media and Diet Trends Be Contributing to a Little-Known Eating Disorder?" *Washington Post,* July 24, 2019, https://wapo.st/2LtYIPN.

4. "Eating Disorder Awareness Week: Eating Disorders by the Numbers," SUNY Broome, February 26, 2018, https://bit.ly /3nMVC6o.

5. Cheyenne Shelby, "The Importance of Wellness," *Muncie Journal,* June 19, 2019, https://bit.ly/3pplHcD.

6. Mary Poplin, "Mother Teresa: Become 'A Pencil in God's Hand,'" Crosswalk.com, February 23, 2009, https://bit.ly/3bMEY4G.

7. Caroline Jones, "Why Is Anorexia on the Rise?" Patient.com, September 21, 2017, https://bit.ly/2LHbSJ1.

8. Cindy Crawford quotation, Instagram, July 24, 2017, https://bit.ly /2LwO76G.

9. Dana Benbow, "Experts: Mom Has Biggest Impact on Girls' Body Image," *USA Today,* August 23, 2013, https://bit.ly/3nTeWic.

Chapter 8: Fight the Good Fight

1. G. K. Chesterton quotation, Twitter, August 17, 2019, https://bit .ly/3qsW0sn.

2. G. K. Chesterton quotation, Twitter, March 25, 2020, https://bit .ly/2YEKyhJ.

3. Jen Pollock Michel, "Learn the Difference Between Right and Almost Right," The Gospel Coalition, October 5, 2018, https:// www.thegospelcoalition.org/reviews/thats-good-recovering-lost -art-discernment.

4. Eric P. Wheeler, *Dorotheos of Gaza: Discourses and Sayings* (Kalamazoo: Cistercian Publications, 1977), 122.

5. C. S. Lewis, *Mere Christianity* (New York: HarperCollins Publishers, 1952, 1980), 121–128.

6. Archimandrite Sophrony, *Wisdom from Mount Athos: The*

Writings of Staretz Silouan (Crestwood: St. Vladimir's Seminary Press, 1974), 87–94.

Chapter 9: Embrace Your Purpose

1. David Uebbing, "Ask Jesus What He Wants and Be Brave, Pope Tells Youth," Catholic News Agency, April 21, 2013, https://bit.ly /2LWgGtW.
2. Rick Warren, *The Purpose Driven Life: What on Earth Am I Here For?* (Grand Rapids: Zondervan, 2012), 18.
3. Emily P. Freeman, "Do the Next Right Thing: A Simple Practice of Making Life Decisions," iBelieve.com, May 3, 2019, https://bit .ly/3qxJAzJ.
4. Father Abbot Tryphon, Ancient Faith Ministries Podcast, "Many Have Contemplated Suicide," March 1, 2001, https:// abbottryphon.com.
5. Christine Caine quotation, Twitter, August 30, 2017, https://bit.ly /3qrG7SZ.

Chapter 10: Live in Hope

1. Helen Keller quotation, Good News Network, June 27, 2020, https://bit.ly/3ba0u0Z.
2. David Mathis, "Made for Another World," Desiring God, November 22, 2016, https://bit.ly/3oSDkSL.
3. Max Lucado, *The Oak Inside the Acorn* (Nashville: Thomas Nelson, 2011), https://amzn.to/2N9wp9z.
4. Elizabeth Bernstein, "An Emotion We All Need More Of," *The Wall Street Journal*, March 21, 2016, https://on.wsj.com /3nMLGtC.

ACKNOWLEDGMENTS

I wrote this book during a global pandemic. Like many moms, I wrestled with burnout, stress, and mental exhaustion during that time.

With my previous books, I knew exactly what to write before I started. This book, however, was different. It required fervent prayer, many calls to trusted friends, and more input from my editors. When my publisher asked for another parenting book, I knew that a mother's well-being (and its ripple effect on the family) should be a central theme, yet I was unsure how to approach this age-old topic in a fresh way.

After all, moms know that we need self-care. We have heard the oxygen mask analogy more times than we can count. What I wanted was a compelling guide to help mothers understand wellness through God's lens. In society today, we tend to either idolize our wellness or neglect it, and I hoped to show a healthy middle ground that leads to peace, purpose, and joy.

I also wanted to offer hope, especially to moms in crisis, and point out that some of our best parenting happens as we face adversity—and what we model for our children through a healthy response.

A big thank-you to the many friends who helped me

brainstorm and nail down the message of this book, especially Mary Alice Fann, Kimberly Powell, Rachel Fry, Shannon Thomas, Alice Churnock, Kim Anderson, Tyler Drouet, and Rebecca Hollingsworth. The title came during a phone call with Rebecca, so I owe a double thanks to you!

To Dr. Michele Borba, one of the smartest and kindest women I know, for your encouragement and long-distance mentoring. Your insights as I started this journey, as you shared the primary struggles you see in your work with mothers and women, solidified the foundation for the heart of this book. I feel lucky to know you and call you a friend!

To my phenomenal editors, Stephanie Newton and Dawn Hollomon, who elevated the manuscript and encouraged me every step of the way. Even on the day my first edits arrived, I received from you a box of delicious cookies and an encouraging note about your belief in this message. Both personally and professionally, you two are a *gift*, and I'm thankful for your patience, kindness, and friendship—as well as your sharp eyes and keen minds as editors. Truly, it is a joy to work with you.

To my agent, Andrew Wolgemuth, whose life illustrates faith in action. Andrew, you show integrity in every email, conversation, and interaction. Your solid judgment, wise counsel, advocacy, and diligence ensure that each book is stewarded well and the right questions get asked. It is an honor to be represented by you and Wolgemuth & Associates.

To the wonderful team at W Publishing Group/Thomas Nelson: Stephanie Newton, Dawn Hollomon, Lauren Bridges, Rachel Guise, Lisa Long, Debbie Wickwire, Damon Reiss, Ashley Reed, Caren Wolfe, Katherine Hudencial, Allison Carter, Hannah Cannon, Kerri Daly, and the marketing and publicity teams. Thank you for making me feel like family. Thank you for keeping this fun and going above and beyond in each collaboration. I can't wait to launch this book with you!

To Father Bob Sullivan, for reviewing the manuscript from a faith perspective and spurring me on. Your imprint on my journey is significant, and your way of drawing hearts to Jesus by succinctly speaking the truth in love is inspirational. Thank you for your life's work and the gift you are to our family and more. We love you!

To the wise women who shared testimonies in this book: Kristin Sartelle, Shannon Thomas, Andrea Goodson, Jill Partridge, Annie Pajcic, Rachel Fry, Meredith Mann, Mary Crenshaw, Whitney Long, and Leann Hanes. Your contributions quickly became my favorite part of this project, and I will read them again and again to remember the big picture. Thank you for sharing your heart and stories. Each reader will be a better person after getting to know you.

To my dad, my biggest fan and faith influence. Thank you for your advice and deep conversations. Thank you for the unconditional love that makes it easy to imagine a loving and merciful heavenly Father. Your children and grandchildren adore you, and we thank God for our Papa who is one of a kind and one of the best humans on the planet.

To my husband, Harry, and our four daughters: Ella, Sophie, Marie Claire, and Camille. My heart bursts with love for you, and you have generated more joy, laughter, satisfaction, hope, meaning, and depth in my life than I deserve. Thank you for supporting me, lifting me, and loving me. It is the greatest privilege to do life with you, and I treasure the family and home life we have built together.

And to Jesus, whose grace is sufficient. I hope I never forget how panicked and mentally blocked I felt when I began this book, because it forced me to depend on you. It erased any illusions of being capable on my own. Each day, you gave me exactly what I needed, and over time those graces added up. Please bless the mothers who read this message. Help them love themselves as a child of God and understand their value through You.

ABOUT THE AUTHOR

Kari Kubiszyn Kampakis is an author, blogger, and national speaker from Birmingham, Alabama. Her bestselling book for moms, *Love Her Well: 10 Ways to Find Joy and Connection with Your Teenage Daughter,* and books for teen girls, *10 Ultimate Truths Girls Should Know* and *Liked: Whose Approval Are You Living For?,* have been used widely across the country for small group studies.

Kari's work has been featured on the *Today* show, *Today Parents,* Focus on the Family, Yahoo! News, Grown & Flown, Thrive Global, Your Teen, For Every Mom, Motherly, FaithGateway, EWTN, Love What Matters, Ann Voskamp's blog, *The Huffington Post,* and other national outlets. She also hosts a podcast called *Girl Mom.* She and her husband, Harry, have four daughters and a dog named Lola. Learn more by visiting www.karikampakis.com or finding Kari on Instagram and Facebook.

10 Ways to Find Joy and Connection with Your Teenage Daughter

For many women, having a baby girl is a dream come true. Yet as a girl grows up, moms hear a disheartening script that treats a teenage daughter's final years at home as solely a season to survive.

Author Kari Kampakis suggests it's time to change that narrative. As a mom of four daughters, she has learned the hard way how to parent from a place of strength and joy instead of defeat and discouragement. By improving the habits and dynamics of the mother-daughter relationship, moms can earn a voice in their teen girls' lives.

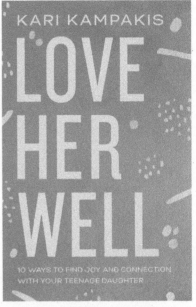

In Love Her Well, Kari shares ten ways that moms can better connect with a teenage daughter in a challenging season, including

- **choosing their words and timing carefully,**
- **listening and empathizing with their teen's world,**
- **being her emotional coach,**
- **taking care of themselves and having a support system, and more.**

Kari gives mothers hope and reminds them all things are possible through God. By leaning on Him, moms will gain the wisdom, guidance, protection, and clarity they need to grow strong relationships with their daughters at every age, especially during the critical teen years.

10 Ultimate Truths Girls Should Know

It's not easy to be a teenage girl. Dealing with cliques, bullying, rejection, and social media fiascos can be overwhelming and disheartening.

Thankfully, there's a way to rise above it. There's a way to find love, acceptance, and security without compromising your integrity, your faith, or your future.

In *10 Ultimate Truths Girls Should Know*, Kari Kampakis offers practical advice, loving support, and insightful discussion questions that will stir your soul and move you to action. As you begin making important decisions about your life, from peer pressure to dating to academics, you can count on this book for guidance and reassurance that God is with you always.

God's plan for you is bigger than you dare to dream. And once you hear His call, only a life with Him will do.

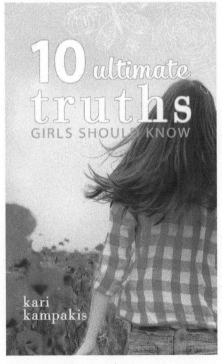

Whose Approval Are You Living For?

For girls growing up in a generation saturated with social media, getting enough "likes," comments, and online friends can become an unhealthy obsession.

With positive and powerful insights, Kari Kampakis encourages girls to apply God's timeless truths in the digital age. Diving deeply into topics like social media, friendship, identity, and faith, *Liked* helps girls think through those questions that may stir wildly in their mind and heart, such as:

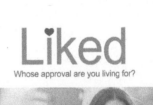

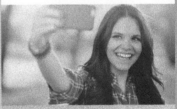

- Who am I?
- What is my purpose?
- How can I change the world and make an eternal difference?
- How can I love myself when I feel unlovable?

For anyone tired of the quest to impress— and ready to rest in God's unconditional love—*Liked* is the answer.